KETO DIET

Simplifying Everything You Need to Know

About Ketogenic Diet For Beginners

CONTENTS

INTRODUCTION

Have you been looking for ways to jump start your health and fitness goals? Are you looking for ways to lose weight and still maintain a healthy body? Well, if that is what you are looking for, then the ketogenic diet is the way to go!

You may have heard of the ketogenic diet and may even be wondering what it is. The truth is, the ketogenic diet is everything you would like to incorporate into your diet routine. It is the ultimate eating plan that will drive your body into ketosis. Ketosis refers to a state where the body uses fats as the primary source of fuel instead of the usual carbohydrates.

When you start consuming the right keto diet we have put together in this book, your body will get you into ketosis within one to three days. One thing that you need to note is that when consuming a keto diet, the majority of the calories that you consume come from fats, a moderate amount of proteins, and minimal carbohydrates.

You may have heard of some claims about the keto diet; "Keto burns fats fast, fights disease or you can eat all the bacon you want to!" In as much as there are lots of celebrity hypes about this diet, the truth is that it is just like any other diet. This is because it requires a gut check!

When you consume your foods in the right proportions, the ketogenic diet will be useful to help lower the risk of certain diseases, boost your weight loss, and keep you in shape. According to research, the keto diet is by far superior to the low-fat diet that is often recommended. In fact, what makes the diet even more useful is the fact that it is filling without necessarily requiring you to count calories in your food intake.

One study demonstrated that people on a keto diet lose at least 2.2 times more weight compared to those that consume a calorie restricted low-fat diet. What is more, the levels of High-Density Lipoproteins (HDL or "good cholesterol") and triglycerides improve. Another study also showed that people on a keto diet lose three times more weight than those on a Diabetes recommended diet.

It is evident that consuming a keto diet will not only help you lose weight, but it will improve your health a great deal. This is because it helps increase the levels of ketones in the body, lower the blood sugar levels, and boosts insulin sensitivity.

It is common knowledge that our body is designed to run on carbohydrates. We use them to provide our body with the energy that is required for normal functioning. However, what many people are clueless about, is that carbs are not the only source of fuel that our bodies can use. Just like they can run on carbs, our bodies can also use fats as an energy source. When we ditch the carbs and focus on providing our bodies with more fat, then we are embarking on the ketogenic train.

Despite what many people think, the ketogenic diet is not just another fad diet. It has been around since 1920 and has resulted in outstanding results and amazingly successful stories. If you are new to the keto world and have no idea what I am talking about, let me simplify this for you.

For you to truly understand what the ketogenic diet is all about and why you should choose to follow it, let me first explain what happens to your body after consuming a carb-loaded meal.

Imagine you have just swallowed a giant bowl of spaghetti. Your tummy is full, your taste buds are satisfied, and your body is provided with much more carbs than necessary. After consumption, your body immediately starts the process of

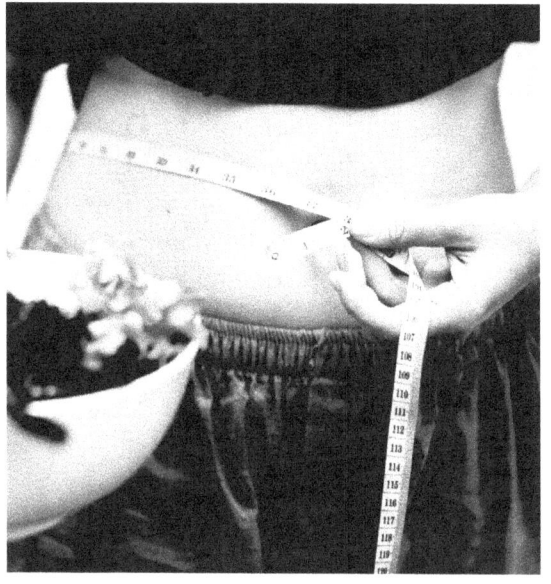

Once your body shifts to using ketones as fuel, you are in the state of ketosis. Ketosis is a metabolic process that may be interpreted as a little 'shock' to your body. However, this is far from dangerous. Every change in life requires adaptation, and so does this.

digestion, during which your body will break down the consumed carbs into glucose, which is a source of energy that your body depends on. One might ask, "what is wrong with carbs?". There are some things. For starters, they raise the blood sugar, they make us fat, and in short, they hurt our overall health. So, how can ketogenic diet help?

Once your liver begins preparing your body for the fuel change, the fat from the liver will start producing ketones – hence the name ketogenic. What glucose is for the carbs, the ketones are for the fat, meaning that they are the tiny molecules that are created once the fat is broken down to be used as energy.

The switch from glucose to ketones is something that has pushed many people away from this diet. Some people consider this to be a dangerous process, but the truth is, your body will run just as efficiently on ketones, as it does on glucose.

Once your body shifts to using ketones as fuel, you are in the state of ketosis. Ketosis is a metabolic process that may be interpreted as a little 'shock'

A ketogenic diet skips this process by lowering the carbohydrate intake and providing high fat and moderate protein levels. Now, since there is no adequate amount of carbs to use as energy, your liver is forced to find the fuel elsewhere. And since your body is packed with lots of fat, the liver starts using these extra levels of fat as an energy source.

to your body. However, this is far from dangerous. Every change in life requires adaptation, and so does this.

This adaptation process is not set in stone, and every person goes through ketosis differently. However, for most people, it takes around two weeks to adapt to the new lifestyle fully

Just remember that this is all biological, and completely normal. You have spent your whole life packing your body with glucose; it is only natural that you also need time to adapt to the new dietary change.

Trust me, these mouth-watering delights are fit for any occasion and eater, you will not believe that these recipes will help you restore your health and slim down your body. Ditching carbs do not mean ditching yummy treats, and with these ingenious recipes, you will see that for yourself.

Successfully practiced for more than nine decades, the ketogenic diet has proven to be the ultimate long-term diet for any person. The restriction list may frighten many, but the truth is, this diet is super adaptable, and the food combinations and tasty meals are pretty endless.

If you require any further information, feel free to contact me: contact@alphaketo.net

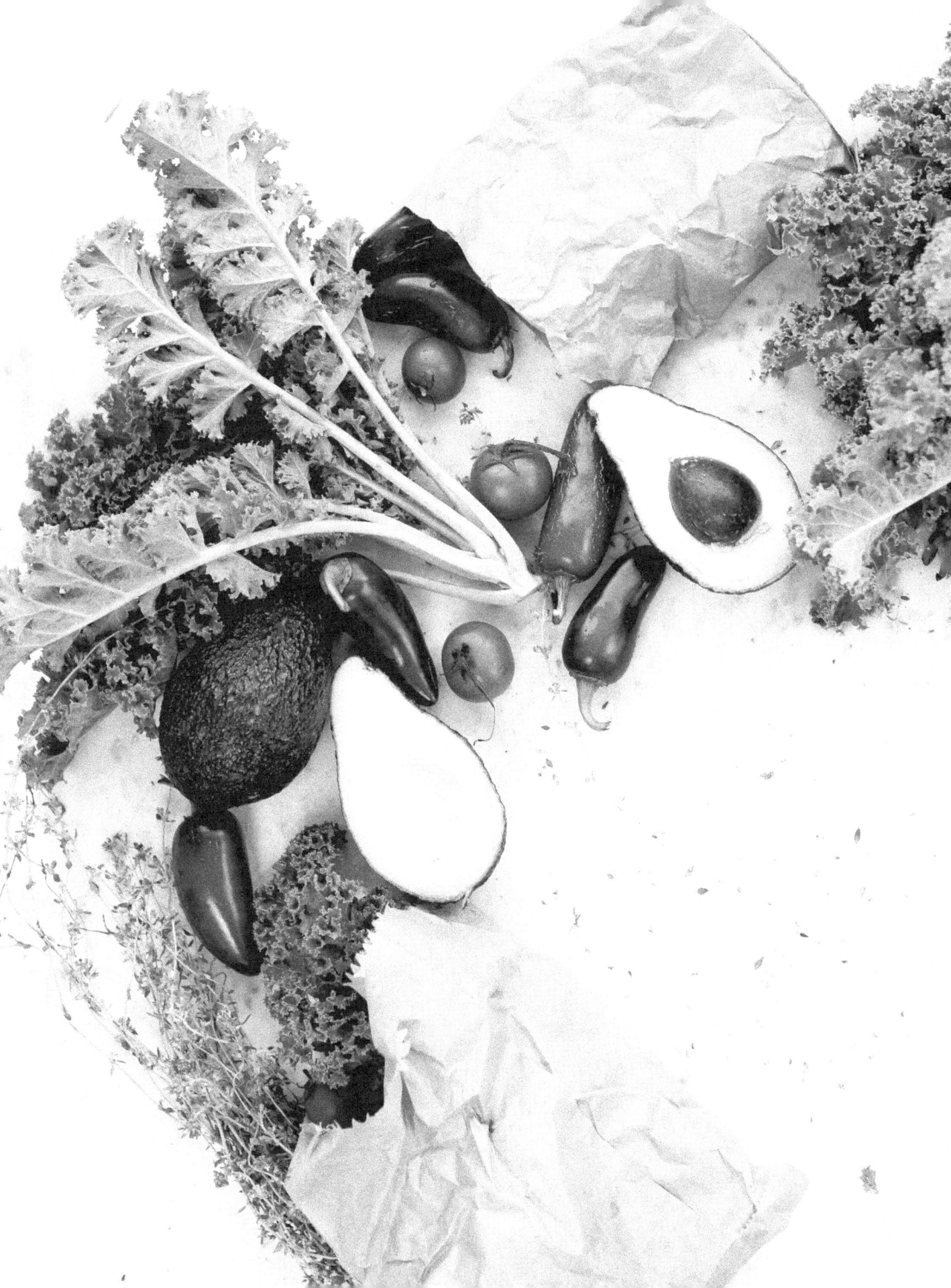

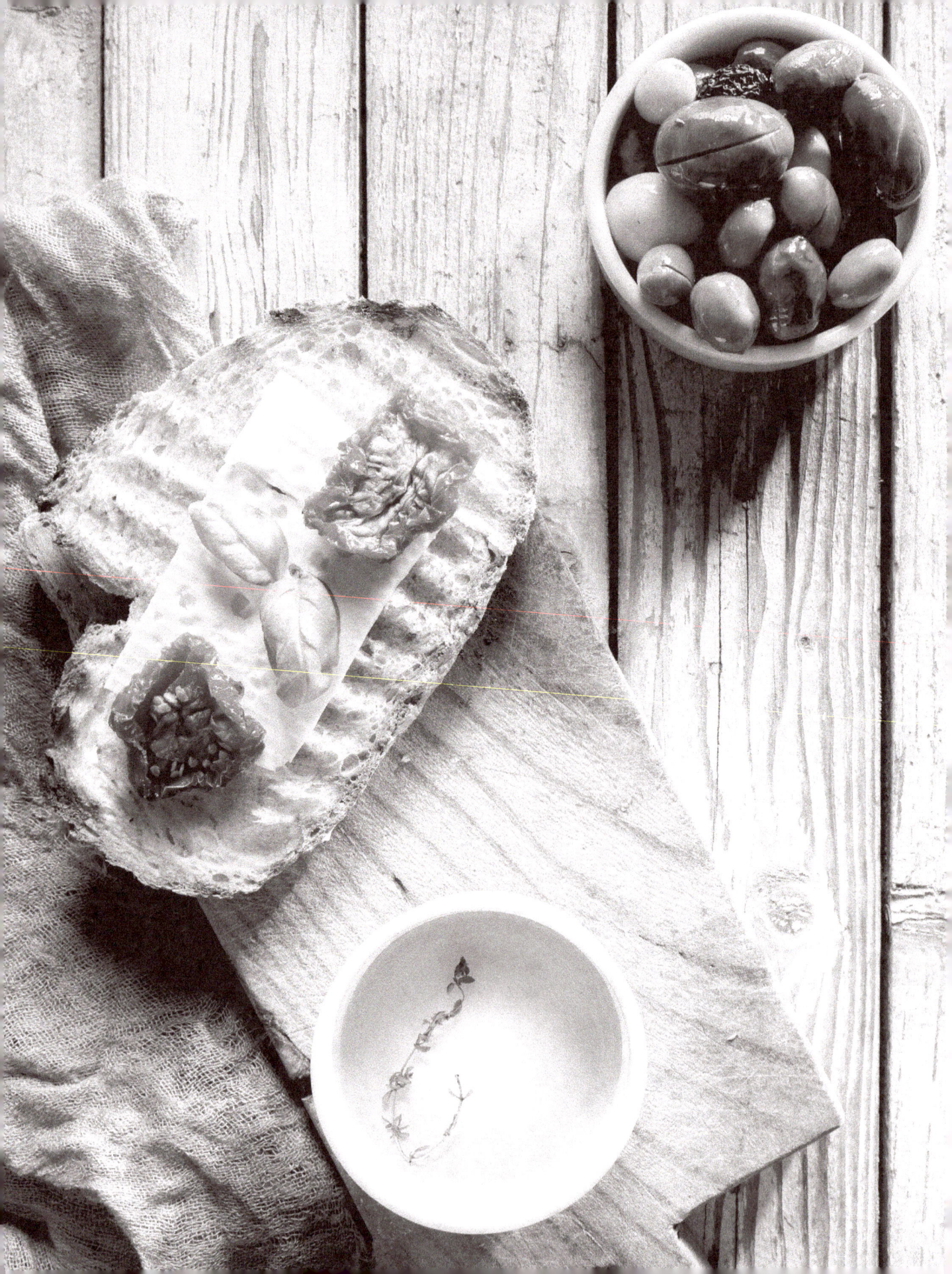

WHAT KETO IS

AND WHY YOU WANT IN ON THE PARTY

What Happens in your Body When You Eat Keto?

One question that I hear so many people asking is; "*What is a keto diet?*" Well, keto comes from the ketogenic diet, which refers to a diet that allows the body to produce small fuel molecules referred to as ketones. In other words, it produces an alternative fuel source for the body, which is used when the levels of sugar in the blood are low.

This is what happens when you are on a keto diet compared to a traditional diet;

When you consume a keto diet, the body produces ketones, which are broken down quickly into blood sugar. When eating a keto diet, you must keep your protein intake at moderate levels. This is because when the protein intake is too high, this can trigger the excess to be converted into blood sugar.

It is the role of the liver to produce ketones from fat. It is these ketones that play a role as a source of fuel throughout the body, and most importantly, for the brain. One thing that you need to understand is that the brain a hungry organ that uses up lots of energy each day.

When on a keto diet, the whole-body switches into fat burning 24/7. However, when the levels of insulin go down, then fat burning has to increase dramatically.

The Keto diet makes it easier to access the fat stores to burn them off, something that is great when you are on a weight loss program.

As the body produces ketones, it enters a metabolic state of ketosis. One of the fastest ways to achieve this state is through fasting. However, no one can fast forever! The good thing with the keto diet is that you can eat it indefinitely and still achieve a state of ketosis.

So, why should you join in on the party?

Well, there are so many health benefits that come from consuming a keto diet. Some of these health benefits include;

Fat burning for weight loss

One thing that I love about consuming a keto diet is the fact that it encourages fat burning. If you are on a weight loss program, then this is what you should start signing up for. It will help you drop those extra pounds pretty fast. This is mainly because when the fats are burned, there follows the production of ketones, which suppress ghrelin - a hunger hormone. At the same time, it boosts the release of cholecystokinin (CCK), which helps you feel full.

When you have a reduced appetite, it merely means that you can go for extended durations of time without having the urge to eat anything. This, in turn, encourages the body to deep into its fat stores for energy.

Reduces the risk of inflammation

According to research, there is evidence that shows that the keto diet has anti-inflammatory properties. This explains the reason why so many people use it to protect against major degenerative diseases like cancer and Alzheimer's among others.

Fuels and feeds the brain

As we have already mentioned earlier, the brain requires lots of energy every day. With ketones, the brain can get an immediate hit of energy of up to 70% of what the brain requires. Fats also feed the brain and help keep it strong.

One important point to note is that the brain is made up of at least 60% fats. This means that it requires lots of good fats for it to keep running. Some of these essential fats include Omega-3, which helps the brain grow and develop. On the other hand, saturated fats go a long way toward keeping the brain's myelin sheath strong so that the neurons can effectively communicate with each other.

The thing with ketosis is that it helps the brain to create lots of mitochondria, which serve as the power generators within the brain cells. When there is more energy produced by the brain cells, this translates to more energy to help you get stuff done.

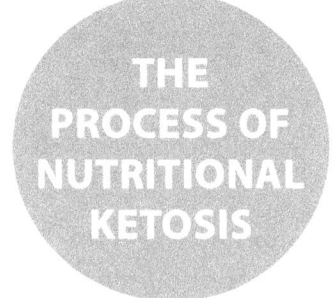

THE PROCESS OF NUTRITIONAL KETOSIS

Carbohydrate intake is decreased.

After the body has used most of its stored glucose, it shifts to using fat for energy.

Dietary fat and stored body fat are broken down for energy, resulting in the production of ketones.

The body also creates glucose from noncarbohydrate sources for the small set of bodily processes that require it.

Ketones become the body's primary fuel, replacing glucose.

Lowers blood sugar levels

Did you know that a keto diet can actually reverse or even cure diabetes? According to research, the keto diet stabilizes the levels of insulin in the body and, in effect, lowers the blood sugar levels. The thing is that the levels of blood sugar are reduced to the point that so many diabetics can come off their medications. The trick is for you to switch to a ketogenic diet!

Unifying Paleo and Low-Carb

It is important to note that as you transition from burning glucose to fat burning, you have to support it with a diet that is loaded with lots of fats. However, this is not completely necessary as you can get into a state of ketosis using several other techniques such as fasting, eating a low-carb/low-fat diet, among others.

From experience, the state of ketosis is best achieved by consuming a whole food-based diet that is high in fats. In other words, what I advocate for you to eat is a high-fat, low-carb paleo diet. Just a minute, I know you must be thinking; "Paleo again? Doesn't that trump low-carbs in so many ways?"

Well, one thing that you have to note is that the Paleo diet prides itself on an abundance of vegetables and fruit, consumption of healthy fats, and a balanced intake of Omega-6 fatty acids. On the other hand, the low-carbs diet is strictly about limiting the number of carbohydrates you take with little to no concern about the quality and sensitivity of the food, something that goes a long way toward contributing to your overall health and diet success. These two phenomena have different viewpoints of the world!

Well, the Paleo diet eliminates sugars and grains. But the truth is that it is lower in carbs than is recommended for a standard American diet. Additionally, the lost amount of carbs are replaced by dietary fats. It is this high-fat, low-carb scenario that has led so many people to believe that these are the key drivers of a successful Paleo diet. Coincidentally, this is on the borderline of nutritional ketosis!

The thing is that people who eat low-carb diets have realized that they can overcome their weight loss plateau quite easy when they increase their fat intake and lower their protein intake simultaneously. Again, this is what the keto diet is about! However, what is interesting is that when the same low-carb eaters go for extended durations of time with minimal carbs, they hit a bumpy plateau spot, have health concerns such as loss of hair, something that can only be remedied by increasing the carb intake.

The approach in the keto diet is to bring the Paleo and low-carb diets together. Therefore, if you are a Paleo advocate, you will derive so much empowerment by simply transitioning into a metabolic state of ketosis based on already balanced primal fare.

The approach in the keto diet is to bring the Paleo and low-carb diets together.

Is Keto Right for You?

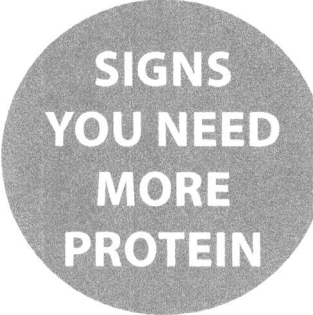

Four criteria will help you know whether the keto diet is right for you. These factors include;

Does it help you meet your body's composition goals?

Let's face it; if you are eating something that is not helping you get the results that you want, then it is high time you started switching things up. If you are consuming a diet to lose weight and you feel that it is not making any difference after a while, then you must make changes that will help you maintain a calorie-deficit.

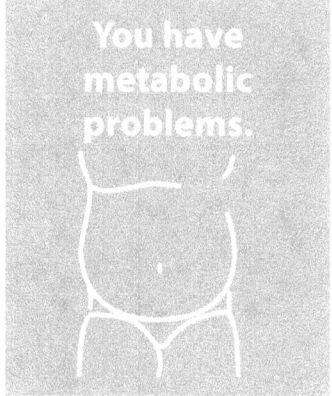

Does it meet your macronutrient needs?

Your diet must have all the right micronutrients in their correct proportions. In other words, your diet has to ensure that you get adequate vitamins, and minerals to maintain optimal health and ward off disease. Even though you can lose your weight without necessarily meeting your micronutrient needs, one thing you will notice is that you will not feel good about it.

Does it improve your overall health and wellbeing?

One thing that people often overlook is the fact that a healthy diet is one that ensures that they not only feel good but also healthy by optimizing various health measures such as bloodwork and body composition among others. If the diet impairs the quality of your life and causes unnecessary suffering and stress, then you must make changes.

That said, although you may feel great on a specific

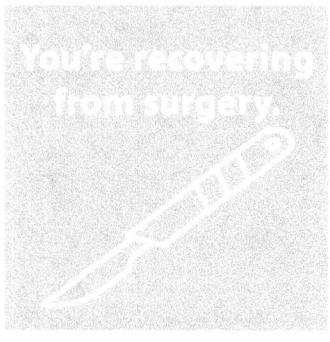

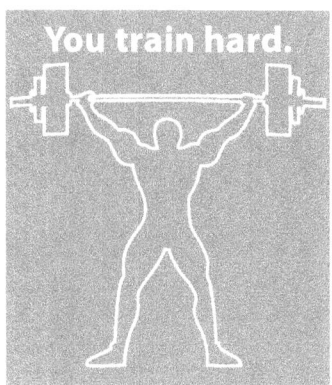

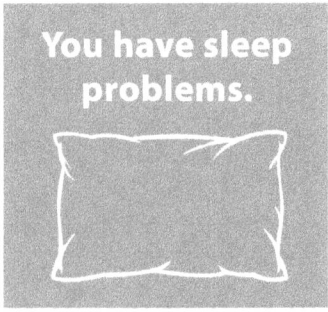

SIGNS YOU NEED MORE PROTEIN

You have sleep problems.

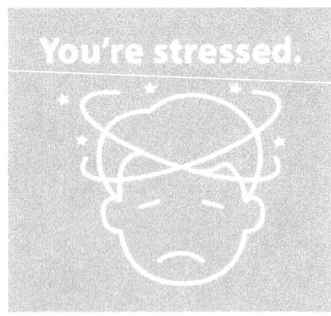

You're stressed.

You're always hungry.

diet, there is a chance that a blood test will indicate that your health is deteriorating. This explains the reason why you should ensure that you keep track of your subjective experience and objective outcomes such as weight, blood sugar levels, waist circumference, and cholesterol levels, among others.

Does it provide you with a dietary approach to use in sustaining your health and wellbeing even in the long-term?

One thing you should note is that any diet can offer you the short-term results that you are looking for. However, the most critical question is to determine whether the diet will maintain your body in the long-term.

The best diet is one that will completely replace your previous eating style and still meet the rest of the criteria we discuss here. If you cannot see yourself sticking to the new diet plan in the long run and are struggling with it in the short term, there is a high chance that you will rebound to your old eating habits and put on more weight.

That said, if you feel that the new diet plan does not fit the four criteria we have discussed irrespective of how much you restrict your carbs and how many ketones you produce, the truth is that your health is likely to suffer. It is therefore crucial that you find out what your ideal optimal diet is and experiment with it. This is important to help you come up with the best dietary strategy that will not only improve your health but will help you accomplish your goals and still sustain the results in the long term.

What about the Cholesterol? And Other Concerns About Eating Fat

Consuming a high fat, low carb diet is incredibly healthy. So many people think that since the keto diet is loaded with high-fat content, they risk raising their blood cholesterol levels. However, one thing that you will notice about the keto diet is that it has potentially life-saving benefits from some of the world's most serious diseases. Some of these include obesity, epilepsy, type 2 diabetes, and metabolic syndrome, among others.

Consuming a low carb diet often lowers the risk of developing heat disease.

Although these risk factors often improve, some individuals experience improvements while others have experienced adverse effects. According to research, there is evidence that shows a small subset of people experience increased levels of cholesterol even on a low carb diet, especially the keto diet and a high-fat version of Paleo.

This often results in an increase in Total

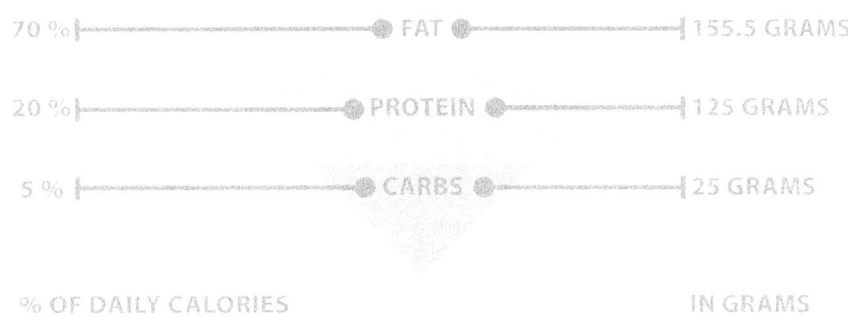

70 %	FAT	155.5 GRAMS
20 %	PROTEIN	125 GRAMS
5 %	CARBS	25 GRAMS
% OF DAILY CALORIES		IN GRAMS

2000-CALORIE DAILY KETOGENIC DIET

cholesterol and Low-density lipoprotein cholesterol. Well, one thing that is important to note is that these risk factors are established in the context of a high carb western diet. What is not known is whether they have a similar effect on a healthy low carb diet that has lower oxidative stress and inflammation.

Check whether you have a family history of heart disease. The good news is that you do not have to eat a very low-fat diet or take statins just so that your cholesterol levels go down. There are simple adjustments that you can make, and you can start reaping all the benefits of consuming a keto diet.

The interpretation of blood cholesterol levels is relatively complex. Most of you are familiar with Total, LDL, and HDL cholesterol. If you have high levels of HDL, then you are said to have a lower risk of developing heart disease. If you have high levels of LDL, the chances are that you will develop heart disease.

However, that is just what we know, right? Well, the real picture is even more complicated than this. The truth is that the bad cholesterol has several subtypes that are classified based on the particle size. People who have small LDL particles often are at a high risk of heart disease compared to those with large particles.

Research shows that the most significant markers of all are the LDL number of particles (LDL-p), and that is important in telling us how many particles are floating in the bloodstream. You should not confuse this with the LDL concentration (LDL-c), which plays a significant role in telling us

how much cholesterol the particles are carrying around in the bloodstream. This is what is measured in a standard blood test.

When you are planning on a new diet, you must get everything checked out so that you know whether there is anything you need to be concerned about. If possible, get your doctor to measure both the LDL-p and the LDL-C. If your cholesterol levels are high, but the LDL-p is normal, then you possibly do not have anything to worry about.

On a keto diet, there is a high tendency for the HDL levels to go up and the triglycerides to go down. At the same time, both the LDL cholesterol and Total cholesterol remain constant. Also, the LDL size often increases, and the LDL-p drops- all the good things! However, this is what happens on average. Within these averages, some experience an increase in cholesterol levels even when on a keto diet.

Well, unfortunately, we cannot all have advanced markers such as ApoB and LDL-p measured. This is mainly because these tests are quite costly and are unavailable in some developing and underdeveloped countries. In such a situation, you can choose to use the Non-HDL cholesterol, which is a reasonably accurate marker used mainly when measuring the standard lipid panel.

If the levels of Non-HDL are high, then this is reason enough for you to start taking precautions in your diet to try and get it down. Therefore, the bottom line is that there are those individuals that experience high cholesterol levels even when they are on a low-carb, high-fat diet (Keto diet).

DIZZINESS / HEADACHES

BRAIN FOG / INSOMNIA

IRRITABILITY

SIMPTOMS
OF KETO FLU

NAUSEA

HEART PALPITATIONS

HYPOGLYCEMIA

DIARRHEA

FATIGUE
MUSCLE CRAMPS

The "Keto Flu"

The keto flue is avoidable and its duration can be reduced simply by adding more sodium to your diet. Here are some of the easiest ways to do it:

◊   Add more salt to your meals.

◊   Drink soup broths like beef and chicken.

◊   Eat saltier foods like pickled vegetables and bacon.

TO REPLACE OTHER ELECTROLYTES, TRY TO EAT MORE OF THE FOODS LISTED BELOW:

ELECTROLYTE	FOODS CONTAINING ELECTROLYTE
POTASSIUM	Avocados, nuts, dark leafy greens such as spinach and kale, salmon, plain yogurt, mushrooms
MAGNESIUM	Nuts, dark chocolate, artichokes, spinach, fish
CALCIUM	Cheeses, leafy greens, broccoli, seafood, almonds
PHOSPHORUS	Meats, cheeses, nuts, seeds, dark chocolate
CHLORIDE	Most vegetables, olives, salt, seaweed

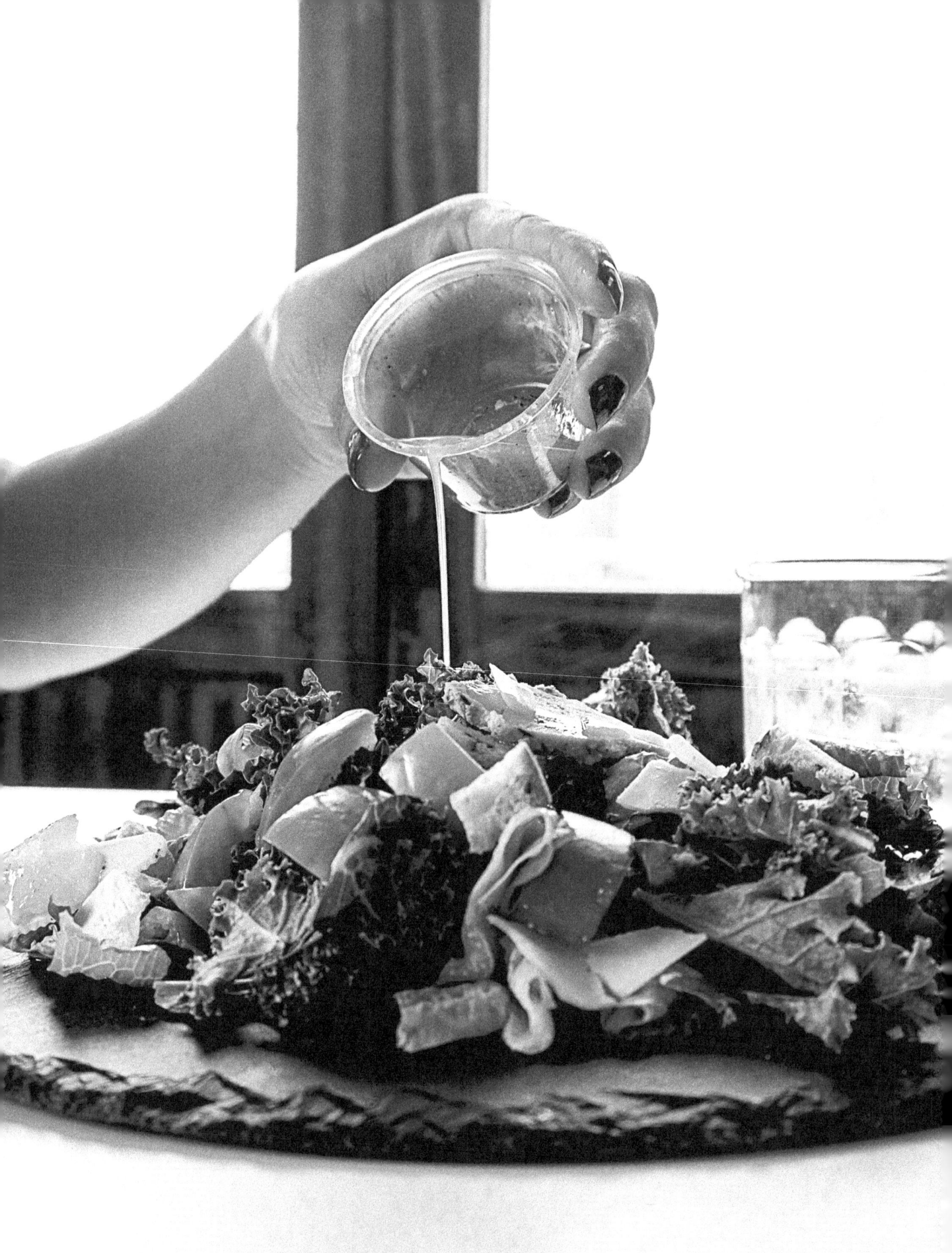

CHAPTER 2

THE KETO EXPERIENCE

How to Know Whether you're in Ketosis

As we have already discussed, ketosis is often termed a metabolic process that takes place when the body starts burning fats for the production of energy. This is mainly because it has low carbs to burn for glucose production. During ketosis, the liver produces chemical particles referred to as ketones.

So, how do you know that you have reached a state of ketosis?

High levels of ketones

When you take a blood sample, there will be an indication of high levels of ketones. This is the most definitive sign of ketosis. Use a ketone testing kit to check the ketone levels at home. You can also use indicator strips to check the urinary levels. When you are in nutritional ketosis, the level of blood ketones will be between 0.5 and 3 millimoles per liter.

Weight loss

According to research, being on a keto diet is effective in ensuring weight loss. This means that if you are on a ketogenic diet, the other sign that you will notice is weight loss. There is evidence that shows that people on a keto diet are likely to shed off a couple of pounds in the long term compared to people on a low-fat diet. This is something that you will be able to observe during the first few days of starting a keto diet. However, actual fat loss may not happen at least until after several weeks.

Headaches

When you are on a keto diet, there is a high chance that you will experience headaches that will last anywhere between a day to a week, or even longer. This often occurs as a result of consuming a low level of carbohydrates, hence dehydration and electrolyte imbalance.

According to recent research, there is evidence that shows that ketogenic diets are a potential treatment for migraines and cluster headaches. For instance, a 2017 study showed that people with episodic and chronic migraines were treated using the keto diet. Another 2018 study suggested that the keto diet is a possible treatment of cluster headaches that were considered drug resistant.

That said, there is a need for further research to confirm how effective the keto diet is in treating or preventing these kinds of headaches. If your headaches persist for longer than a week, you must seek medical advice.

Thirst

When you enter a state of ketosis, the chances are that you will feel thirstier than usual. This is mainly because you are losing water as a side effect of consuming a keto diet. However, you also ought to realize that when the levels of ketones are high in the body, there is a high chance that you will feel dehydrated and experience an electrolyte imbalance.

These two effects may be accompanied by severe complications such as kidney stones. To avoid this from happening, it is essential that you take plenty of water and other non-sugary fluids. However, if dehydration symptoms persist, you should seek medical advice.

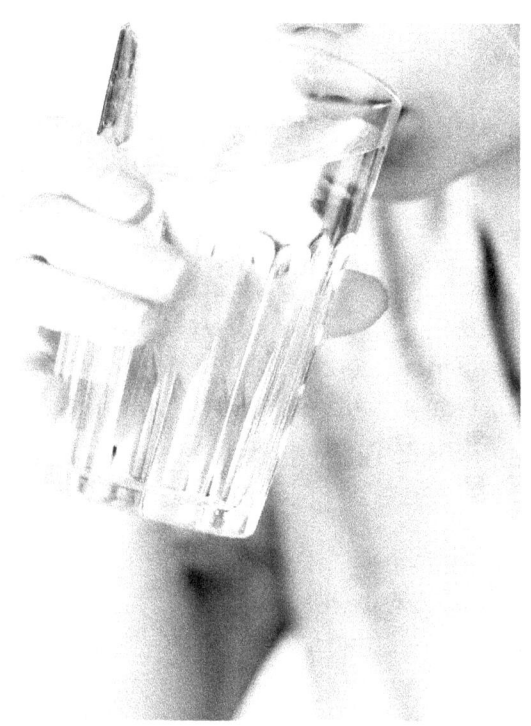

Muscle cramps and spasms

One of the effects of dehydration and electrolyte imbalance is muscle cramps. It is the role of the electrolytes to transmit electrical signals between various cells in the body. When there is an imbalance, this can disrupt electrical messages, causing muscle contractions and spasms.

When you are on a ketogenic diet, it is highly likely that you will experience muscle cramps and spasms from an electrolyte imbalance. However, you can counter these effects by ensuring that you consume foods that are rich in electrolytes. Some of the most essential electrolytes in the body include magnesium, sodium, calcium, and potassium.

You can get sufficient quantities in your balanced diet. However, if symptoms persist, you can make dietary changes or take supplements.

Fatigue and weakness

During the initial stages of consuming a keto diet, you may experience fatigue and general body weakness. This often is a common occurrence when your body switches from carb burning to fat burning for energy. Carbs are known to provide a faster energy boost to the body compared to fats.

A study conducted in 2017 demonstrated that athletes on a keto diet experience fatigue as a common side effect of the keto diet. This is something that the participants observed during the first two weeks of initiating the diet.

After several weeks on a keto diet, you should start experiencing a burst of energy. If not, then you must seek medical attention. This is because fatigue may be associated with several other factors, such as dehydration and nutrient deficiencies.

Stomach complaints

When you make dietary changes, there is an increased risk of digestive complaints or stomach upsets. This is typical to those getting started on a keto diet.

To lower the risk of these complaints, it is advisable that you drink plenty of water and other fluids. In fact, you can eat plenty of non-starchy vegetables and fiber-rich foods to lower the occurrence of constipation. You could also consider taking probiotic supplements for a healthy gut.

Sleep changes

When you start following a keto diet, you are likely to experience disruptions in your sleep patterns. At first, you may experience difficulties falling asleep. This kind of symptom will typically go away within just a few weeks.

Bad breath

This is a common side effect of ketosis. This is mainly because when you are in a state of ketosis, there is an accumulation of ketones in the body, and they leave the body through urine. People on this diet often have a breath that smells sweet or fruity.

This is because a ketone referred to as acetone is responsible for the odor. However, other ketones such as acetophenone and benzophenone also are likely to contribute to this bad breath. Well, there is no definite way to lower occurrence of ketosis breath as it will improve over time. However, you may want to use sugar-free gum or brush your teeth several times throughout the day to help mask the smell.

As we have already discussed, ketosis is often termed a metabolic process that takes place when the body starts burning fats for the production of energy.

Better focus and concentration

When you get started on a keto diet, you will experience headaches which may get in the way of your attention span. However, with time, these symptoms begin to fade away. If you continue the diet in the long term, you will start experiencing better focus and clarity of thinking.

In fact, according to a 2018 systematic review, epileptic patients following a ketogenic diet were shown to have better attention and alertness as evidenced in their cognitive tests.

Other studies have also shown that taking a keto diet, in the long term, enhances neuroprotective effects and cognitive function.

What to Expect When You Go Keto

If you are thinking of getting started on a keto diet, here some of the things that you need to prepare for;

You will enter a state of ketosis

The main aim of consuming a keto diet is so that you can enter a state of ketosis. This means that your body will start burning fats instead of carbs for energy production. It is expected that you transition into ketosis within 24-48 hours after consuming a keto diet. However, this depends on the number of carbs you intake.

Well, some people have the wrong impression of keto diets. They think it is that diet in which you avoid grains and sugar! In reality, the keto diet requires that you also forgo fruits, legumes, most dairy products, and starchy vegetables for you to hit low-carb targets.

You may feel awful at first: keto flu

You may have heard all the amazing stories that people give about consuming a keto diet. However, all these amazing things do not just happen out of the blue. At first, you will experience keto flu. Well, this is less of a sickness and more of a type of lethargy. The truth is that the body often prefers to source its energy from carbs. Therefore, when it makes that transition into fat burning for energy, the body is not able to supply the required amount of energy as fast. This kind of feeling brings about the keto flu, which lingers for a week or until the body can adjust fully. Therefore, you should adapt into your diet gradually to make the transition smooth for the body.

You will need to adjust your workouts

Remember what we said about the body preferring to run on carbs? Well, one thing that you will realize is that consuming a keto diet will have adverse effects on your workout sessions at first. This is because the body is still trying to adjust to a new energy source, and hence, you will feel fatigued and weak to do any exercise.

Therefore, try to pause your workout plan at least for the first few weeks after getting started on a keto diet. Once your body is entirely in ketosis and is well adjusted, you can resume your workouts as usual.

Your gut may be off

According to a survey, there is evidence that shows most Americans do not get an adequate supply of fiber to begin with. This is often the case before cutting out such fiber-rich foods like whole grains, beans, veggies, and fruits as is required by a keto diet.

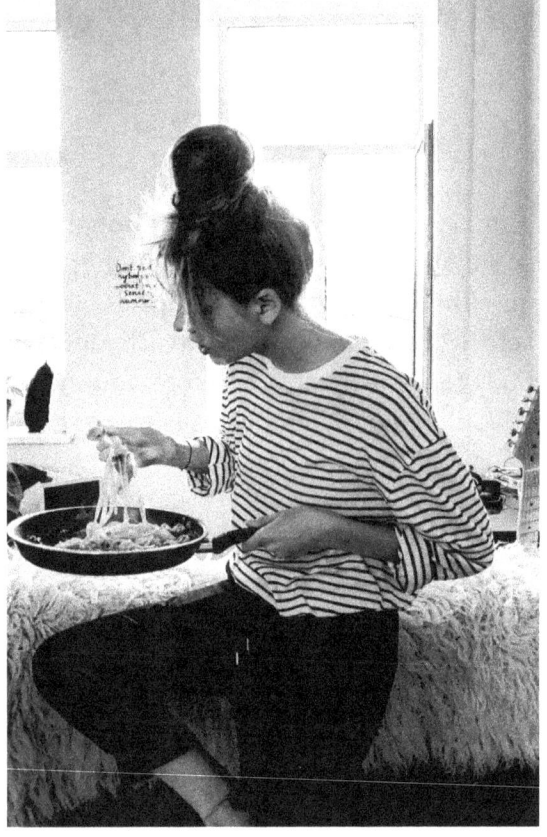

You will not have the same reaction to keto as your friend

When starting off on a new diet, it is easy to compare what you are experiencing with what your friend, neighbor, or coworker is feeling. Although you may be on the same diet, you will not feel the same with anyone else, for that matter.

Some will tell you that being on the keto diet has made them feel better and have more clarity than they have ever had in their life. However, you may be experiencing quite the opposite. You should not compare yourself with your colleagues. However, you can check in with them to try and adjust where necessary.

The best thing is for you to work closely with a dietitian who will be able to help you plan your diet better before you can get started on a keto diet. It is also critical that you ensure what you eat makes you feel great. If being on a keto diet makes your days more a slog and you feel very miserable about it, then this may not be the right diet for you.

You may want to eat a lot

When you hear the term diet, the first thing that might come to mind is going hungry. While the keto diet is restrictive, it is mostly composed of loads of fats. The good thing about consuming fats is that they are satiating. When I first got started on the keto diet, I was surprised at how satiating it was. You may be thinking how tough it is to eat fats throughout the day, and yes, it might take some effort before your daily intake is perfect.

This is a fair warning!

When you are on a keto diet, the main focus is on fats and meats, which are not loaded with fiber. This makes it quite easy to miss out on foods that are important for digestion. Cutting down on fiber-rich foods often contributes to constipation. Irrespective of what your diet is, the main aim should be to keep the fiber as low as 25 and 30 grams for women and men, respectively.

To counter the effects of constipation, it is advisable that you eat such foods as greens, avocados, and broccoli, among others. It is also essential that you take plenty of water and up your levels of activity.

Food to Eat

The plan is simple, cut down on carbohydrates and increase all healthy fats while keeping the rest of your diet the same. This may sound easy, but when you look for foods with little to no carbs, the list is short and perplexing—a mix of some vegetables, fruit, and meat. Here are all the appropriate foods to take on a low carb keto diet:

- Vegetables are grown above-ground, including cauliflower, zucchini, broccoli, etc.
- Everything green, including spinach, kale, etc.
- Seeds and nuts, including pistachios, sunflower seeds, pumpkin seeds, almonds, etc.
- Berries and avocados
- Low-carb sweeteners including Stevia, monk fruits, and erythritol.
- Dairy and plant-based fats, including cheese, butter, olive oil, coconut oil, etc.

Food to Avoid

All high-carb ingredients are strictly prohibited on the ketogenic diet. For processed products, make sure to read the labels and check the level of carbs in them. Generally, the following ingredients should be crossed off from your grocery list while on the ketogenic diet.

- Legumes such as; lentils, chickpeas, all forms of beans, etc.
- Grains such as; wheat, cereals, rice, corn, etc.
- All forms of sugars, maple syrup, agave, honey, etc.
- Tubers such as yams and potatoes
- Fruits like bananas, pineapples, watermelons, oranges and apples, etc.

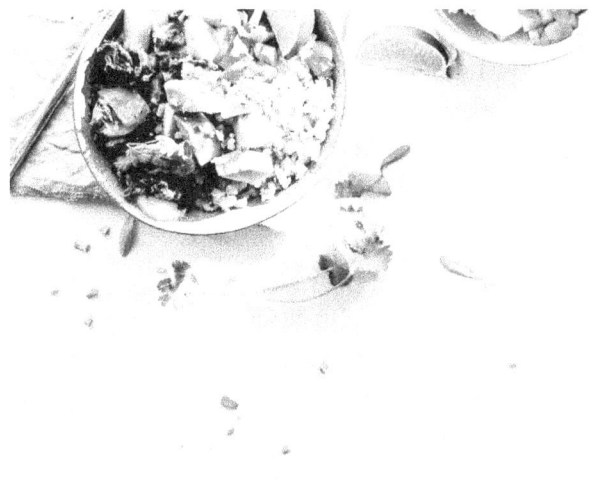
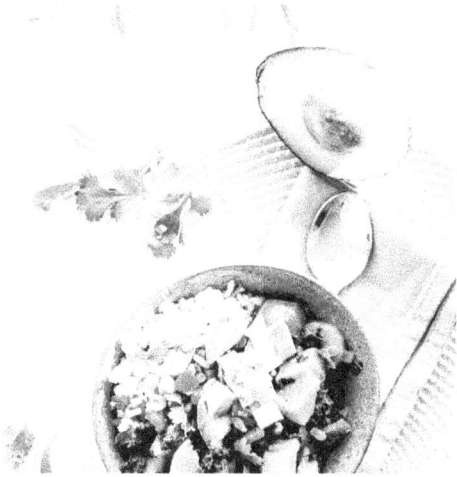

Common Mistakes for Beginners

There are quite several mistakes people make when getting started on a keto diet. Some of these mistakes include;

Mistake #1
Using a keto diet as a quick fix

So many people try to use the keto diet as a quick fix for their body issues. One thing that you need to note is that keto diets are not your quick fix. Instead, it is a lifestyle change that you need to stick to in the long-term.

You will notice some changes relatively fast. However, this does not mean that you can jump right back into your old eating habits and still expect to see the change you are looking for. Trust me. If you do this, you will fall back into your old ways so fast it will make your head spin!

Well, when on a keto diet, there are times when you can slip back from the plan just for a little bit, and you can slip right back, and that is alright. The truth is that there is nothing that is going to be permanently different when you stick to a keto diet for several months. So, bear in mind that this is a lifestyle change that you need to stick to in the long-term.

Mistake #2
Obsessing over the scale

Indeed, the keto diet is designed to help you shed some body fat. However, the first thing that you need to accept is that this is a process that takes time, hard work, and discipline. Therefore, obsessing over your weight is not going to make things happen in a split second but only make things harder than they already are.

But what does it mean to obsess over the scale? This is you checking your weight several times a day. When you do this, you are only letting negativity get into your head, and things will begin to go south for you. The best thing you need to do is to trust the whole process and dedicate yourself to do everything the right way. This means staying away from sugars and carbs. That way, your weight is going to come off.

If you keep checking your weight every hour, you will end up getting discouraged. You have to notice that there is no massive change in weight that can happen in hours. A significant change is an accumulation of small changes over several days, weeks, and months. Not hours! The best option is for you to check your weight only once a week and then keeping the same time every week.

Mistake #3
Being afraid of fats

For a very long time, people have been told that fats are very bad for you. However, with the keto diet, you must eat fats to lose fats. When you calculate your macros, you

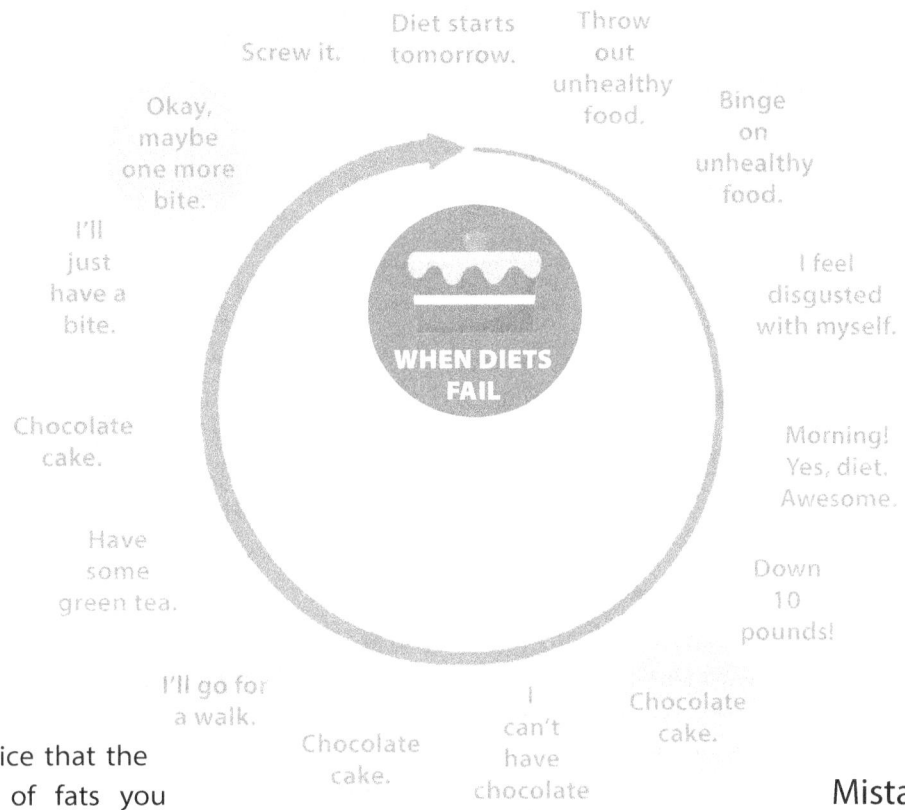

Diet starts tomorrow.

Screw it.

Throw out unhealthy food.

Okay, maybe one more bite.

Binge on unhealthy food.

I'll just have a bite.

I feel disgusted with myself.

WHEN DIETS FAIL

Chocolate cake.

Morning! Yes, diet. Awesome.

Have some green tea.

Down 10 pounds!

I'll go for a walk.

I can't have chocolate cake.

Chocolate cake.

Chocolate cake.

may notice that the amount of fats you have to consume is massive. When you are on a keto diet, you must increase your fat intake so that your body can realize the goals you are striving to achieve.

One thing that you need to understand is that the food you eat on a keto diet needs to be composed of 75% fats. This may come as a shock to you. However, if you are going to be successful in this diet, you will need to keep things this way. Therefore, you should not be afraid of the amount of fats you have to consume. Understand that the keto diet is eventually going to help only if you stick to it and follow everything as it is presented to you. This way, you will not face any more problems.

Mistake #4
Consuming the wrong fats

Yes, we have mentioned that the keto diet is about consuming 75% fats in the diet. However, this does not mean that you should consume all sorts of fats. You must consume the right fats. Do not just assume that because you get the recommended daily fat requirements, you are eating the right types of fats. Bear in mind that there are good and bad fats.

Some of the bad fats that most people struggle with are the processed ones. These are often found in vegetable oil, and this means that you should avoid cooking using these oils. The best fats that you need to incorporate in your keto diet are saturated fats, monounsaturated and polyunsaturated fats, and trans fats, which are naturally occurring.

When you are trying hard to avoid all processed fats, you must consume these good fats. You can find them loaded in eggs, walnuts, avocados, butter, and fish oils, among other sources. You can also get them from fat bombs. These sources will offer you the fats you are desperately looking for when you are on a keto diet. So, add them to your meals and watch how you quickly hit your daily fat requirements while still consuming good fats.

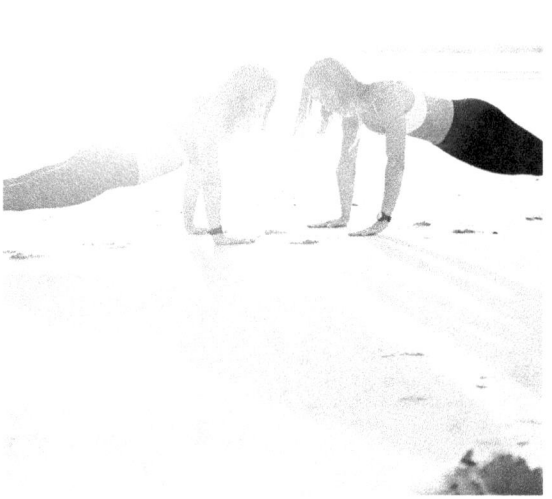

Mistake #5
Eating too many proteins

To many people, this might not seem like a bad thing at all. You are not allowed to consume so many carbs, and therefore, the best way to supplement that is by eating proteins. However, the first thing that you have to notice is that consuming too many proteins has adverse effects on the body when you are on a keto diet.

You have to notice that the body requires a moderate amount of proteins and anything more than that gets converted into fats. What we are trying to do on a keto diet is eliminate body fats and therefore, anything that is trying to add more fats back in is negative.

To counter this, you have to pay close attention to the number of macros you consume.

You must stay with your macros and all else will fall back in place. This way, you will not need to worry so much about having excesses. All you have is just what you need.

Mistake #6
Comparing yourself to others

This is something that many people do not realize is holding them back from achieving their diet goals. You may not even notice it because it is all in mind. Yes, comparing yourself to others is part of humanity. However, when you keep doing it on a keto diet, you may end up getting discouraged.

We cannot all respond to diet changes the same way, and we will not hit milestones at the same time as others.

Some see changes quickly while others will go through the process slowly. This means that you have to understand yourself and pay attention to you alone and nobody else.

Your friend may lose weight faster than you and, if anything, you should be the first one to congratulate them so that they can also encourage you to keep going. You have to understand that your weight loss is happening and though at a slow rate, you will eventually reach your goals. Do not give up. Keep going, and finally, everything will fall into place.

Mistake #7
Not getting an adequate amount of sleep

The process of ketosis can often trigger the body to losing a bit of sleep, especially once the body starts using fats as a source of energy. Therefore, there is a need for you to try as much as you can to get an adequate amount of sleep. We all need the right amount of sleep to get the body functioning well.

When you fail to get the right amount of sleep, the chances are that your body functions will be impaired. So, get adequate sleep so that the body is better equipped to handle changes that come along with consuming a keto diet.

Mistake #8
Not taking enough water

When you are on a keto diet, one thing you will notice is that your body will lose a lot of fluids. This means that you have to replenish them by drinking lots of water to stay hydrated as much as possible. Unfortunately, this is something that most people seem to forget.

You are losing lots of fluids and electrolytes, and if you do not get it right back where it needs to be, then there will be an imbalance. Additionally, this kind of imbalance often encourages as much fat storage as possible, something that is the opposite of what we would like to achieve.

By staying hydrated, you are ensuring that your body organs function as they should. The body will function like a well-oiled machine. Yes, you may not be used to drinking lots of water regularly or throughout the day. However, I realize that it is something that needs to be done! The recommended amount of water for an average adult per day is a gallon. Sounds a lot, right? But if you take a few sips here and there throughout the day, you will achieve this target.

Mistake #9 - Not mixing up meals

When on a keto diet, the first thing that you will note is that you are restricted on the number of carbs you take in and you may start thinking that the restriction is also on the number of recipes you use. Because of this, you may end up eating the same meal over and over again.

Well, if you are doing this because you only like a specific type of food, then it is understandable. However, when you start mixing things up, you will begin enjoying this diet plan a whole lot more. It is by having a different meal every other time that your morale will start to go up and allow you to stick to the keto diet in the long-term.

Also, remember to add in some low-carb veggies, because not all recipes will include vegetables. Trust me, when you keep your taste buds guessing, you will enjoy your diet, and your food will not start to taste bland when you keep eating things regularly. There is nothing worse than eating your favorite meal all the time, and before long you get sick of it because you have had too much of it.

Can I Work Out on the Keto Diet?

Well, the most straightforward answer to this question is: YES! Well, of course, we have mentioned that when you are getting started on a keto diet, there is the tendency for energy levels to run low as the body tries to adjust to burning fats for energy from what it is used to (carbs for energy). However, this does not mean that exercise is entirely off-limits. One thing that you need to realize is that working out plays a critical role in helping you lower the risk of heart disease, diabetes, and obesity, among other conditions.

However, it is critical that you exercise care when choosing the type of exercise to engage in. It is even advisable that you seek the doctor's, nutritionist, or certified trainer's advice to ensure that you are participating in workout exercise that goes along with a keto diet.

The keto diet affects your performance when working out. In other words, when you get started on a keto diet, you may not be able to work out as intensely or as often as you did before. Here are some of the most important factors to consider before you engage in workout exercise while on keto.

Factor 1: Ensure that you are eating enough

This does not mean taking enough calories; it means ensuring that you are consuming healthy fats. Workouts often utilize carbs faster than any other macronutrient. Fats are commonly consumed later during workouts. This means that if you are not taking adequate nutrition, it will be quite challenging to sustain a simple exercise. You are risking putting yourself in danger.

Factor 2: Avoid high-intensity workouts

One thing that is important to bear in mind is that more is not always the better option. This is especially the case when you are on a keto diet. Workouts often rely on carbs that have been stored away, something that you will not have when following a

The keto diet affects your performance when working out. In other words, when you get started on a keto diet, you may not be able to work out as intensely or as often as you did before.

keto diet. Therefore, you must stick to a low-intensity workout, most notably during the very first few weeks of introducing the new keto diet.

Factor 3: Listen carefully to your body

When getting started on a keto diet, you must listen to your body carefully. Try not to push yourself too hard when your body is trying to tell you that it cannot handle it. When you have ongoing feelings of fatigue, exhaustion, and dizziness, they could mean that your body is not responding well to the keto diet, and that includes workouts.

Realize that the keto diet can exert so much pressure and stress on the body, something that might take several weeks to adjust fully. Therefore, do not push yourself too hard just because you want to lose weight. If you do pace yourself, then you must ensure you eat well. Also, ensure that you listen to your feelings; mental, physical, and emotional.

	AEROBIC EXERCISE	ANAEROBIC EXERCISE
Activities	Distance running, cycling, dancing, cross-country, skiing, swimming	Sprinting (cycling or running), weight training, high.inensity interval training
Duration	Sustained for long periods	Short, high-intensity sessions
Primary benefits	Strenghtens lungs and heart	Builds strenght and muscle mass
Fuel source	Carbs(glucose/glycogen) or fat	Carbs (glucose/glycogen)

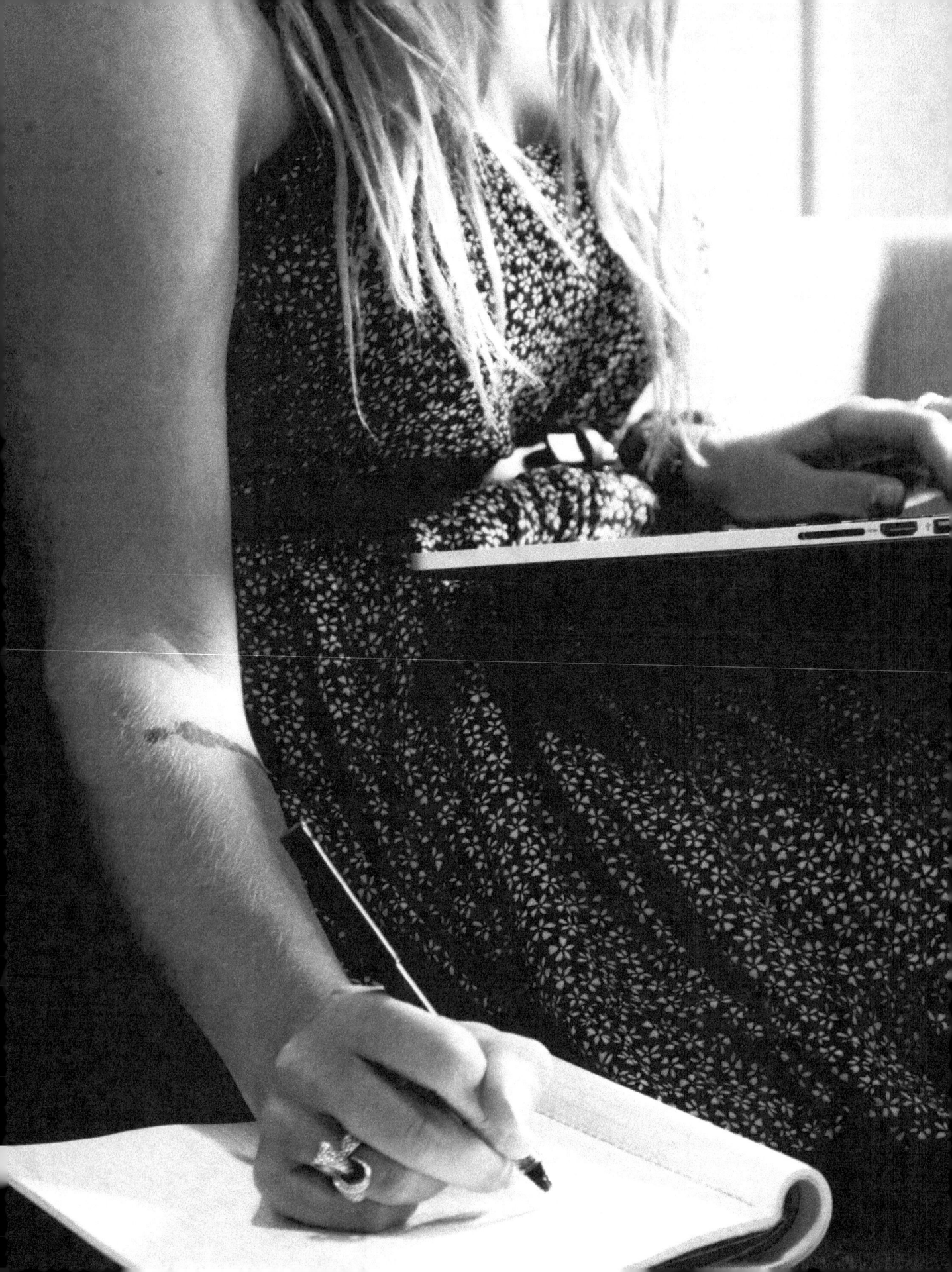

CHAPTER 3

HOW TO
GET STARTED

Steps to take before beginning the Keto Diet

There are steps that you need to take before you can get started on a keto diet. These steps include;

Step #1 Know the foods you will eat and avoid when on a keto diet

A keto diet involves severely limiting the amount of carbs that you consume. Therefore, you must start with about 20 grams of carbs/day and work your way to bringing it down to even as low as 15 grams.

Additionally, you must know what foods are loaded with carbs, fats, and proteins. This will help you to make the right choices. You may be thinking that just bread, cookies, pasta, ice cream, and chips are loaded with carbs. However, beans are rich in carbs and proteins. Fruit and veggies, on the other hand, are loaded with carbs. Therefore, when you know what foods contain which nutrients, you will be better placed to stick to the right foods for your keto diet.

Step #2 Examine your relationship with fats

Note that the keto diet contains lots of fats. Preparing for a high-fat diet can be uncomfortable at first. However, if you start making small adjustments to what to eat each day, you will eventually have it right.

In other words, rather than ordering potatoes or rice with your meals, you can opt for non-starchy vegetables instead. Also, you can start cooking with edible oils. Understand that making a plain skinless grilled chicken breast will not make so much sense on a keto diet as this will not offer you the required daily dietary fats your body needs. Therefore, start introducing lots of healthy fats into your diet and cut out carbs. If you are scared of fats, then the keto diet is not for you!

Step #3 Hone your cooking skills

This is one of the most important things that you need to do before getting started on a keto diet. This is mainly because you want to make something fresh and healthy every day. Here, we have prepared a list of breakfast, lunch, and dinner recipes that you can use when you are on a keto diet. If you are going to stick to the plan in the long-term, then you had better start enjoying cooking in the first place. Otherwise, foods might get boring soon and cause you to go back to your old eating habits.

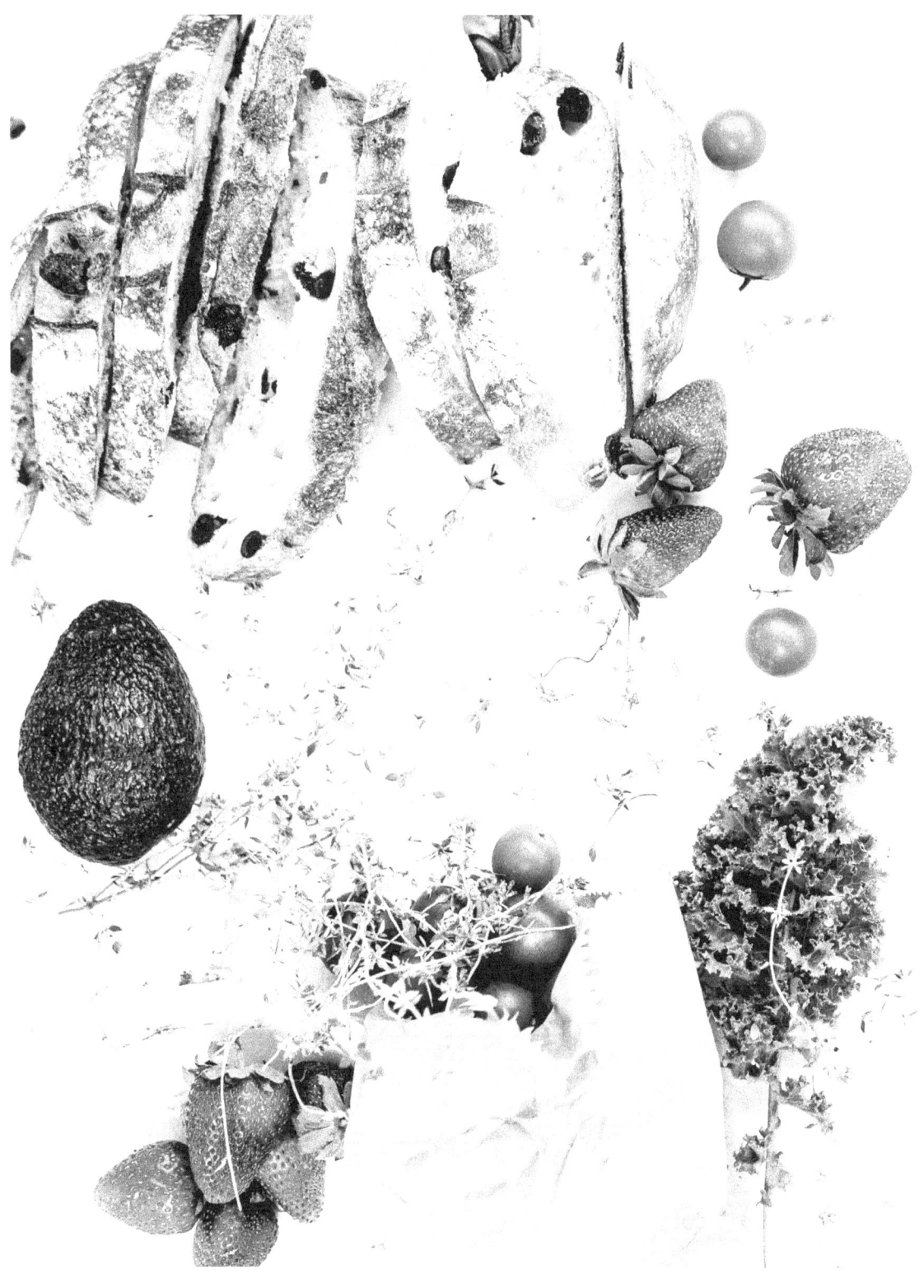

Step #4 Try taking bulletproof coffee

This is one of the best keto-friendly drinks of all time. It is prepared by simply mixing butter and coconut oil into your coffee. This drink will not only keep your hunger at bay but will also offer you an adequate amount of time to plan on what your next meal will be.

However, one thing that is important to note is that coconut oil has the potential of increasing the LDL levels in the body. Therefore, if you have a history of heart disease, this may not be the best option for you.

If you do not know whether you have risk factors for heart disease, be sure to check with your doctor first before taking this drink.

Step #5 Fill your family in on your weight loss goals

The first people who are going to support you through this journey are your family. It is therefore crucial that you let them know you are on a keto diet and would like to lose weight.

This will ensure that they support you when they are eating non-keto meals during family mealtimes.

Assure them that this is only temporary and soon you will be able to get back to normal. If they try to push you, the best thing is to let them know that you have done your research well and know that it is safe, and you want to do it. Be strong.

Step #6 Beware of the side effects such as keto flu

One of the most significant side effects that you need to be aware of before getting started on a keto diet is the keto flu. This does not mean that there are no other side effects, but this is the most serious one.

The keto flu often refers to the duration soon after starting the keto diet, and your body has not fully adjusted to burning fats for energy. Some people have no problem with this, while some become miserable.

During the first few days, your limbs may be feeling extremely lethargic, and climbing up the stairs may become impossible. You also may have to deal with a severe mental fog. For these reasons, you must select a start date during a week when your schedule is not crazy with so many obligations and deadlines to meet.

In other words, choose a time that is slow and when you have an adequate amount of time to rest. Also, try to take it easy on workouts during the first weeks at least until your body has fully adjusted to burning fats for energy rather than carbs for fuel.

Step #7 - Up your electrolyte intake/balance

This goes a long way toward helping mitigate the unpleasant side effects of being on a keto diet. Understand that during ketosis, the kidneys often excrete lots of electrolytes and water. Staying dehydrated can contribute to further complications in your health. That way, it is critical that you take in adequate amounts of minerals;

potassium, sodium, and magnesium among others to help the body function optimally. The best way to do this is to salt your food, eat non-starchy veggies, and drink salted bone broths, among others.

Step #8 Have an after the plan

After you have achieved your goals, what next? Well, this is a question that most people don't get to figure out when getting started on a keto diet. However, one thing that you need to remember is that the keto diet is not a long-term weight loss solution. You will not be on keto forever because it is designed for use in the short-term.

Rather than going back to your old eating habits after achieving your weight loss goals on keto, you must shift your diet into a healthy pattern that will ensure that you keep that weight off in the long run. Otherwise, you risk putting on the weight you have lost and lost all the health benefits you gained.

Therefore, before you start, take time to think about how things will be once your keto diet time is over. Ask yourself how you intend to use this temporary diet as a springboard to improve your health in the long term.

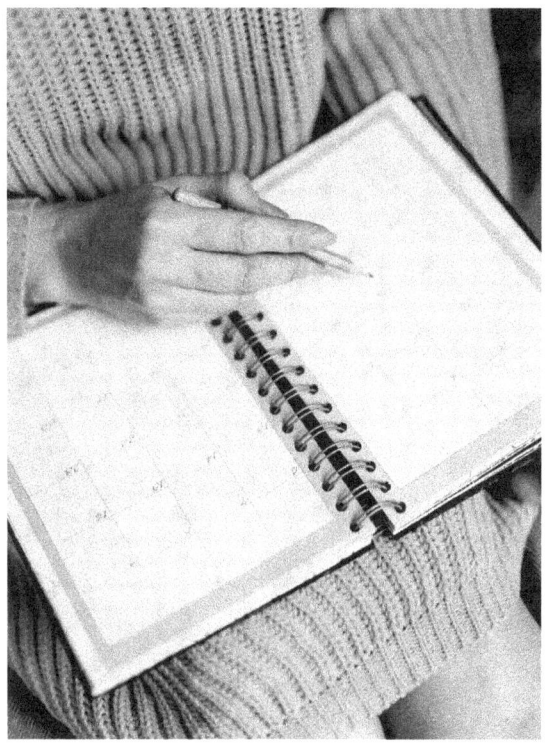

Here, we have prepared a list of breakfast, lunch, and dinner recipes that you can use when you are on a keto diet. If you are going to stick to the plan in the long-term, then you had better start enjoying cooking in the first place.

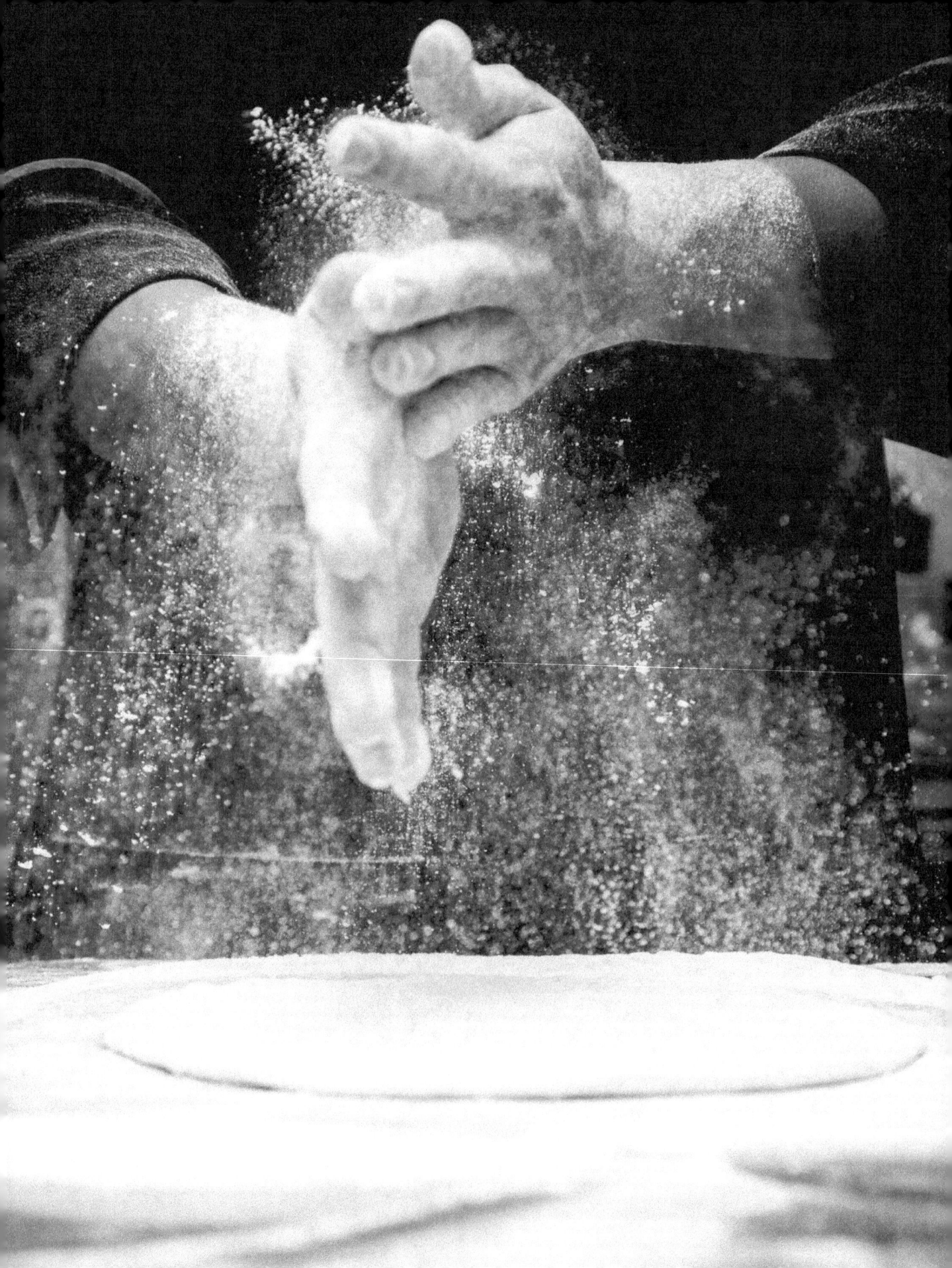

CHAPTER 4

FREQUENTLY ASKED QUESTIONS AND ANSWERS ABOUT KETO DIET

Question 1
WHAT IS A KETO DIET?

Well, a keto diet is very low-carb, a high-fat diet that triggers a metabolic state of lipolysis, where the fats are burned for fuel rather than carbs. The product of this process is particles referred to as ketones, which are used as an energy source by the body.

Question 2
ISN'T THE KETO DIET JUST ANOTHER DIET FAD?

Well, that is not the case! The keto diet is real. It is a lifestyle change that cannot be used as a temporary fix to your body issues. It has been shown to effectively help in sustaining weight loss and providing several other health benefits in the long term.

Question 3
WHAT ARE THE HEALTH BENEFITS OF CONSUMING A KETO DIET?

Some of the benefits you will enjoy from consuming a keto diet include;
* *Weight loss*, which in effect lowers the risk of several other diseases such as heart disease, stroke, type 2 diabetes, cancer, autoimmune diseases, joint problems, premature death, and reduced quality of life among other complications.
* Reduced visceral fats
* Stabilizes blood sugar levels
* Maintains a healthy blood pressure level

Question 4
I HAVE READ THAT KETOSIS IS DANGEROUS, IS THIS A FACT OR JUST ANOTHER MYTH?

It is quite unfortunate that most people confuse ketosis for ketoacidosis. One thing you need to understand is that ketosis is harmless and is a fundamental metabolic process. Ketoacidosis, on the other hand, is a dangerous condition that often is associated with uncontrolled diabetes.

Question 5
ARE THERE SIDE EFFECTS OF CUTTING OUT CARBS?

Well, some people often experience diarrheas and digestion problems. The good thing is that these side effects clear away within a couple of weeks of starting a keto diet. Therefore, it is vital that during these first few days, you increase your intake of high-fiber non-starchy veggies such as leafy greens and broccoli, which help a great deal in alleviating constipation and supplements such electrolytes as magnesium.

Question 6
WILL I HAVE TO GIVE UP ALCOHOL WHEN ON A KETO DIET?

It is important to note that when you drink alcohol, the body will have to burn that for fuel. This means that once alcohol is burned for fuel, fats will not be burned. While this may not stop weight loss altogether, it delays the process. This is mainly because the body does not store alcohol in the form of glycogen. The breakdown of fats will resume after all the alcohol has been broken down.

However, you have to note that alcohol often interferes with weight loss. If this is not a problem for you, then you can take alcohol sparingly. It is also essential that you choose the right type of alcohol, which is not full of carbs or sugars. Bear in mind that alcohol is just full of empty calories, and if you are on a keto diet, you should choose what is most important to you; your weight loss goals, or enjoyment that lasts for a moment.

Question 7
DO I HAVE TO COUNT MY CALORIES WHEN ON A KETO DIET?

Well, the simple answer is no! When you are on a keto diet, you should eat to your satisfaction hence no need to count calories. When you have already eliminated the unhealthy fats and carbs from your diet, you are better placed to keep your cravings in check.

The most important thing is for you to pay attention to what your body needs and only eat when you are hungry. This means that you can skip meals if you feel full. This may be tough for some people. However, you have to realize that when the body burns fats in place of carbs, you will have adequate energy without necessarily feeling the need to replenish it every few hours.

Question 8
IS THE KETO DIET RIGHT FOR EVERYONE?

Well, this diet is ideal for people who would like to lose weight, are struggling with such health conditions as diabetes, or would like to lower their risk of developing heart disease, type 2 diabetes and many more chronic conditions. Notice that the keto diet is different for each individual. Therefore, you must experiment to find out if it works well for you. It is also recommended that you seek your doctor's advice before you get started on a keto diet.

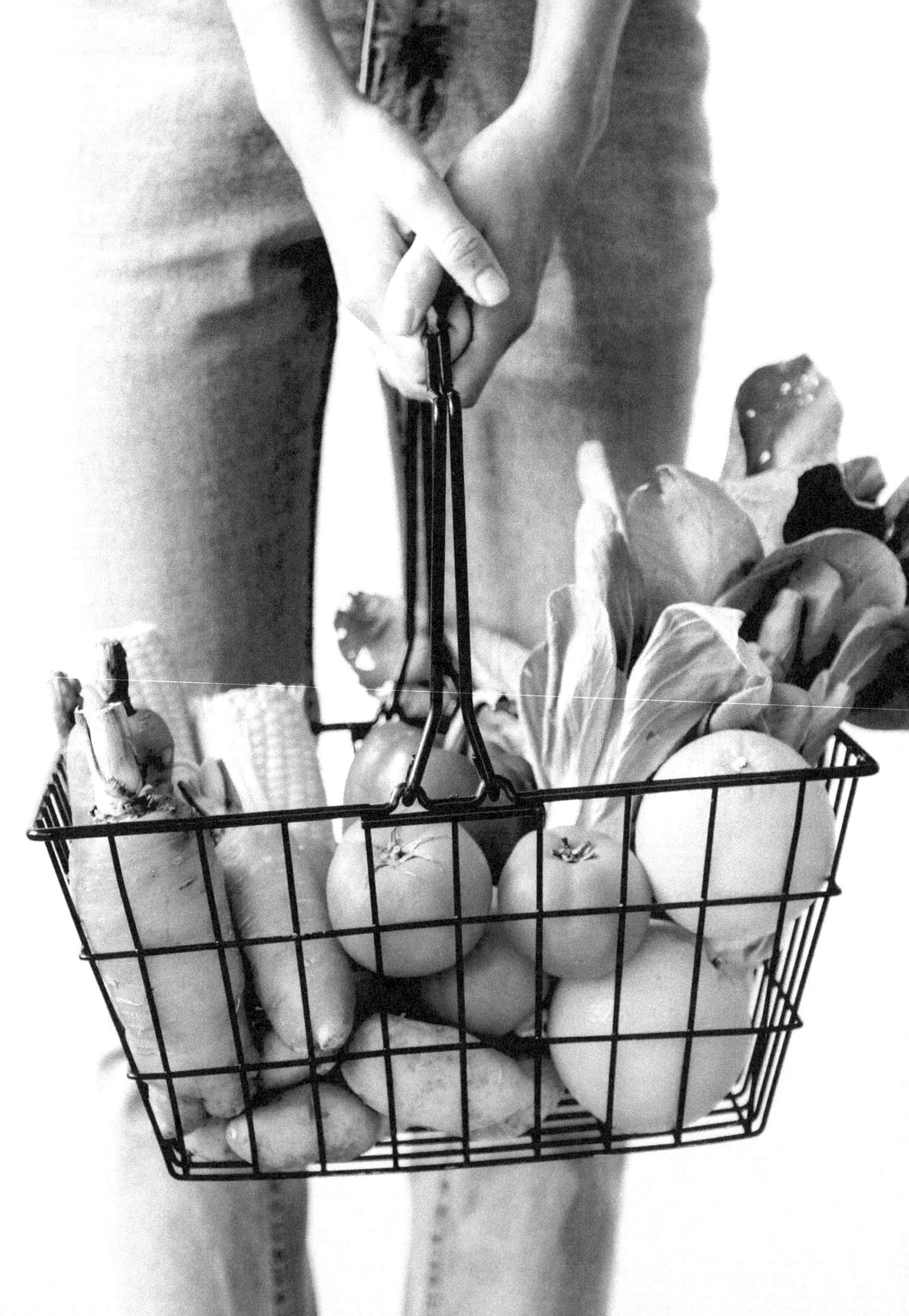

CHAPTER 5

MEAL PLANS
AND SHOPPING LISTS

7 Day Keto Meal Plan

Day 1
Breakfast
Savory Zucchini Muffins
Lunch
Seared Tuna Steak
Dinner
Oven-Baked Chicken in Garlic Butter
Snack
Keto Hoagie Biscuits

Day 2
Breakfast
Breakfast Sausage Patties
Lunch
Easy Stir Fry Kimchi & Pork Belly
Dinner
Cheesy Chicken and Rice
Snack
Green tea mug cake

Day 3
Breakfast
Breakfast Pockets
Lunch
Crispy Baked Fish Sticks
Dinner
Chicken with Cauliflower Rice
Snack
Salmon and Cream Cheese Bites

Day 4
Breakfast
Savory Zucchini Muffins
Lunch
Seared tuna steak
Dinner
Oven baked chicken in garlic butter
Snack
Green tea mug cake

Day 5
Breakfast
Blackberry scones
Lunch
Spicy baked chicken
Dinner
Chicken with cauliflower rice
Snack
Keto Hoagie Biscuits

Day 6
Breakfast
Keto eggcups
Lunch
Bacon-wrapped pork chops
Dinner
Baked meatballs
Snack
Green tea mug cake

Day 7
Breakfast
Coconut macadamia bars
Lunch
Garlic butter steak

Dinner
Low carb chicken skillet
Snack
Blackberry Nut Fat Bombs

Shopping List For 7 Day's Meal Plan

ITEM	QTY	ITEM	QTY
Eggs	115	Asparagus	3.5 lbs.
Egg whites	4	Half and half	1/4 cup
Green onion	2 cups	Artichoke hearts	2 cups
Cheddar cheese	8 cups	Coconut flour	1/2 cup
Can Tomatoes	1/4 cup	Pumpkin puree	1/2 cup
Spinach	22 oz	Ground pork	1 lb.
Coconut milk	2 cup	Cabbage head	1
Zucchini	5	Shrimp	4.5 lb.
Ham	8 oz.	Avocado	1
Roasted Red pepper	15 oz.	Chicken breast	14lbs
Pesto sauce	1/4 cup	Sour cream	1 cup
Parmesan cheese	2.5 oz	Mayonnaise	4 cup
Italian sausage	1 lb.	Bacon	1/2 cup
Almond flour	11 cup	Carrots	6
Erythritol	1 cup	Celery	3 cup
Blueberries	1/2 cup	Salsa	12.5 oz.
Bananas	3	Pepper jack cheese	5 oz.
Walnuts	1 1/2 cup	Almonds	1/4 cup
Jalapeno chilies	3	Cranberries	1/4 cup
Parmesan cheese	1 1/4 cup	Cauliflower	5
Coconut flour	1/3 cup	Pumpkin	1/4 cup
Can Tomatoes	63 oz.	Cream cheese	9 oz.
Kale	1 cup	Baby carrots	5
Chives	1/4 cup	Ground beef	3 lbs.
Feta cheese	1 1/4 cup	Chicken thigh	1 1/2 lbs.
Olives	1 1/2 cup	Swiss cheese	5 oz.
Cherry tomatoes	4 cup	Bell pepper	1/2 cup
Tomato	8	Salmon fillets	8 lbs.
Serrano chili pepper	1	Pork chops	4
Cilantro	2 tbsp.	Chuck roast	2 lbs.
Broccoli	8 cups	Sun-dried tomatoes	1/2 cup
Mushrooms	35 oz.	Chicken	2 lbs.
Cottage cheese	18 cup	Capers	5 oz.
Mozzarella cheese	3 cup	Halibut fish fillets	4
Almond milk	1 cup		
Cauliflower rice	12 oz.		
Onion	10		

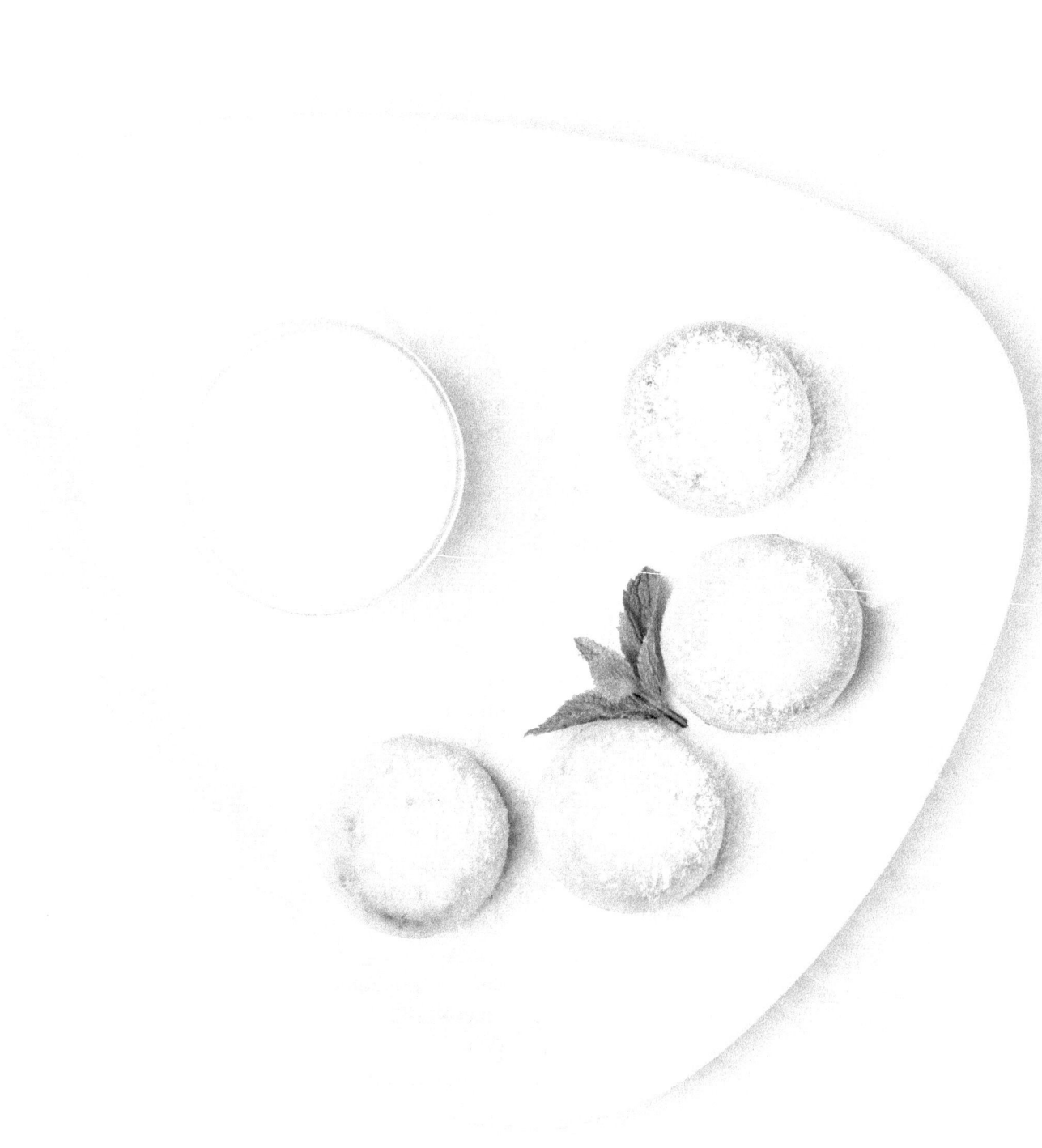

CHAPTER 6

KETO DIET
BREAKFAST RECIPES

BREAKFAST SAUSAGE PATTIES

Serves 8 *Prep Time:* 5 minutes *Cook Time:* 10 minutes *Total time:* 15 minutes

Ingredients
- ✓ 1 tablespoon olive oil
- ✓ 1/4 teaspoon red pepper flakes
- ✓ 1 teaspoon salt
- ✓ 1 teaspoon garlic powder
- ✓ 1 teaspoon dried sage
- ✓ 1 teaspoon fennel seeds
- ✓ 1 pound ground pork

Directions
1. Mix the pork along with the seasonings in a small bowl. Mix until well incorporated.
2. Get 3 tablespoons of the mixture and make equal sized balls using a cookie scoop. Flatten the balls using your hands to form 1/2 inch thick patties.
3. Over medium high heat, heat a heavy bottom skillet or a cast iron and then add in olive oil to coat.
4. Add in the patties and cook them for approximately 5 minutes per side, or until brown. (The internal temperatures should reach 165 degrees)
5. Drain the patties on a paper towel and serve. You can also freeze the patties raw for about 6 months. When you want to eat them, simply defrost and cook normally.

Nutritional information per serving:
Calories 131, Carbs 1.2g, Protein 22.9g, Fat 14.13g

SAVORY ZUCCHINI MUFFINS

Serves 10 **Prep Time:** *20 minutes* **Cook Time:** *25 minutes* **Total time:** *45 minutes*

Ingredients
- ✓ 1/4 cup water
- ✓ 1/4 cup heavy whipping cream
- ✓ 4 large eggs
- ✓ 1 1/2 teaspoons baking powder
- ✓ 1/4 teaspoon black pepper, ground
- ✓ 1/2 teaspoon pink Himalayan salt
- ✓ 1 tablespoon dried Italian herbs
- ✓ 1/2 teaspoon garlic powder
- ✓ 2 teaspoons onion powder
- ✓ 1/2 cup grated Parmesan cheese
- ✓ 4 tablespoons flax meal
- ✓ 1 cup almond flour
- ✓ 1 cup grated cheddar cheese
- ✓ 1 medium zucchini, grated
- ✓ 6 large slices raw bacon

Directions
1. Preheat the oven to 350 degrees F/ then cook the bacon until crispy.
2. Cut the cooked bacon into thin strips and put them in a pan. Add in 1/2 cup water and cook on medium heat for about 10 to 15 minutes, or until crispy.
3. Grate cheddar and zucchini and set aside.
4. Mix all the dry ingredients in a bowl.
5. Whisk cream, eggs and water in a different bowl; and then add in the mixture with the dry ingredients.
6. Blend well and add the new mixture to the crisped up bacon, grated cheddar and the grated zucchini.
7. Mix and then spoon the batter into muffin cups. Put the cups in the preheated oven and bake until the muffin tops are brown, or for 15 to 30 minutes.
8. Remove from the oven and allow to cool for about 5 minutes. Serve or store the muffins in an airtight container in the fridge for up to 5 days.

Nutritional information per serving:
Calories 215, Carbs 5g, Protein 12.7g, Fat 16.6 grams

BREAKFAST POCKETS

Serves 8 *Prep Time:* 15 minutes *Cook Time:* 20 minutes *Total Time:* 35 minutes

Ingredients

Dough:
- ✓ 1 teaspoon salt
- ✓ 2 teaspoons baking powder
- ✓ 1 egg
- ✓ 1/3 cup coconut flour
- ✓ 2/3 cup almond flour
- ✓ 2 oz cream cheese
- ✓ 8 oz mozzarella cheese shredded or cubed

Filling Ingredients:
- ✓ 1/2 cup cheddar cheese, shredded
- ✓ 4 oz Canadian bacon, cooked
- ✓ 2 eggs scrambled

Directions

1. Preheat the oven to 350 degrees F. Meanwhile put the cream cheese and mozzarella into a heat safe bowl and microwave for 60 seconds.
2. Stir and microwave again for 30 seconds. Stir again and check if the cheese has melted. Microwave for yet another 30 seconds or until the cheese resembles a fondue.
3. Into a food processor, add in the melted cheese mixture and the rest of the dough ingredients and pulse until you get uniform dough. You can also knead the dough as well.
4. Divide the firm dough into 8 portions and press individual pieces into 6-inch circle on a baking sheet lined with parchment paper.
5. Divide the filling between individual dough circles and fold in the edge. Crimp to seal well and then put onto the parchment with the seam side down.
6. Bake the pockets until golden brown, or for approximately 20 to 25 minutes.
7. Serve immediately or you could also let them cool and put them in a plastic baggie and freeze. To serve, simply microwave them for 90 seconds and enjoy.

Nutritional information per serving:
Calories 258, Carbs 6g, Protein 16g, Fat 18g.

KETO EGG CUPS

Serves *12*   ***Prep Time:*** *10 minutes*   ***Cook Time:*** *20 minutes*   ***Total Time:*** *30 minutes*

Ingredients

- ✓ Salt and pepper
- ✓ 12 eggs, beaten
- ✓ Filling Options:
- ✓ When it comes to filling options, you have 5 options to choose from!
- ✓ Cooked chorizo+ Monterrey Jack cheese+ minced jalapeño+ cherry tomatoes+ diced avocado
- ✓ Cooked sliced mushrooms + gruyere+ caramelized onion+ chive
- ✓ Mozzarella + Baby tomatoes + basil
- ✓ Turkey + cherry tomatoes + shredded spinach + cooked crumbled bacon
- ✓ Ham + white cheddar + cooked chopped asparagus + baby peas + cooked leeks

Directions

1. Preheat your oven to 350 degrees F. Meanwhile grease 12 muffin cups and set aside.
2. Line the muffin cups with deli meat, and then add in cooked meats or cooked veggies.
3. Beat eggs in a bowl, season with pepper and salt, and then pour the mixture into the muffin tins to the top.
4. Top with cheese and bake until the muffins are puffed and are set in the middle when jigged, or for about 18 to 20 minutes.

Nutritional information per serving:
Calories: 144, Carbs 1g, Protein: 17g, Fat: 29g

BLACKBERRY SCONES

Serves 6   *Prep Time:* 10 minutes   *Cook Time:* 20 minutes   *Total Time:* 30 minutes

Ingredients

For the keto blackberry scones
- 170 g blackberries fresh or frozen
- 7 tablespoons coconut oil
- 1/2 teaspoon kosher salt
- 1 teaspoon xanthan gum or 1 tablespoon flaxseed meal
- 3 1/2 teaspoons baking powder
- 3-5 tablespoons erythritol xylitol, or other sweetener
- 20g whey protein isolate or more almond flour
- 60g psyllium husk or golden flaxseed meal,

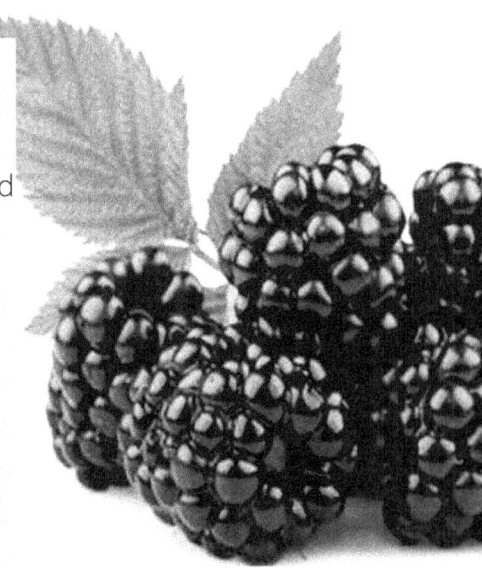

- finely ground
- 96g almond flour
- zest of 1 freshly grated lemon
- 2 teaspoons vanilla extract
- 1 tablespoon apple cider vinegar
- 77g sour cream or coconut cream + 1 tablespoon vinegar
- 1 egg

For the lemon glaze
- 1-3 teaspoons lemon juice as needed
- Zest 1/2 lemon
- 3-6 tablespoons powdered xylitol or erythritol
- 21g coconut flour

Directions

1. Preheat your oven to 450 degrees F and then line a baking stray with a baking mat or parchment paper.
2. Add coconut cream or sour cream, egg, vanilla extract, apple cider vinegar and lemon zest into a medium bowl and whisk the mixture until fully blended. Set aside.
3. Add in flaxseed meal, almond flour, whey protein, coconut flour, xanthan gum, baking powder, salt and sweetener of choice to a food processor.
4. Pulse the mixture until fully incorporated. Now add in coconut oil and pulse for a number of times until its pea-sized.

5. Pour in sour cream and egg mixture and pulse until blended. Lightly flour the baking tray with some coconut flour and dump the dough.
6. With your hands, fold in the blueberries and form the mixture into a circle. Cut the dough into 6 wedges using a knife, and separate them to give room while baking.
7. Brush the dough with melted butter and bake until deep golden, or for 15 to 20 minutes. Let the scones cool down for about 10 minutes.
8. Meanwhile start preparing the lemon glaze. Mix the lemon zest with the sweetener and continue to add lemon juice as required until you achieve the required consistency.
9. Store the blackberry scones in an airtight container for approximately 3 to 4 days, at room temperature not frozen. You can also freeze raw scones for a month or so then bake them straight from the freezer when needed.

Nutritional information per serving:
Calories 320, Carbs 11g, Protein 7g, Fat 29g

COCONUT MACADAMIA BARS

Serves 6   ***Prep Time:*** *5 minutes*   ***Total Time:*** *5 minutes*

Ingredients
- ✓ 20 drops stevia drops
- ✓ 6 tablespoons shredded coconut, unsweetened
- ✓ 1/4 cup coconut oil
- ✓ 1/2 cup almond butter
- ✓ ½ cup macadamia nuts

Directions
1. First crush the macadamia by either hand or using a food processor.
2. Mix the shredded coconut, coconut oil and almond butter in a mixing bowl. Add in the crushed nuts along with stevia drops.
3. Mix the ingredients until well blended and then pour the batter into a 9 by 9-baking dish, lined with parchment papers.
4. Keep the bars refrigerated, preferably overnight. To get crunchier breakfast bars, put them in the freezer.

Nutritional information per serving:
Calories 327, Carbs 7g, Protein 5g, Fat 33g

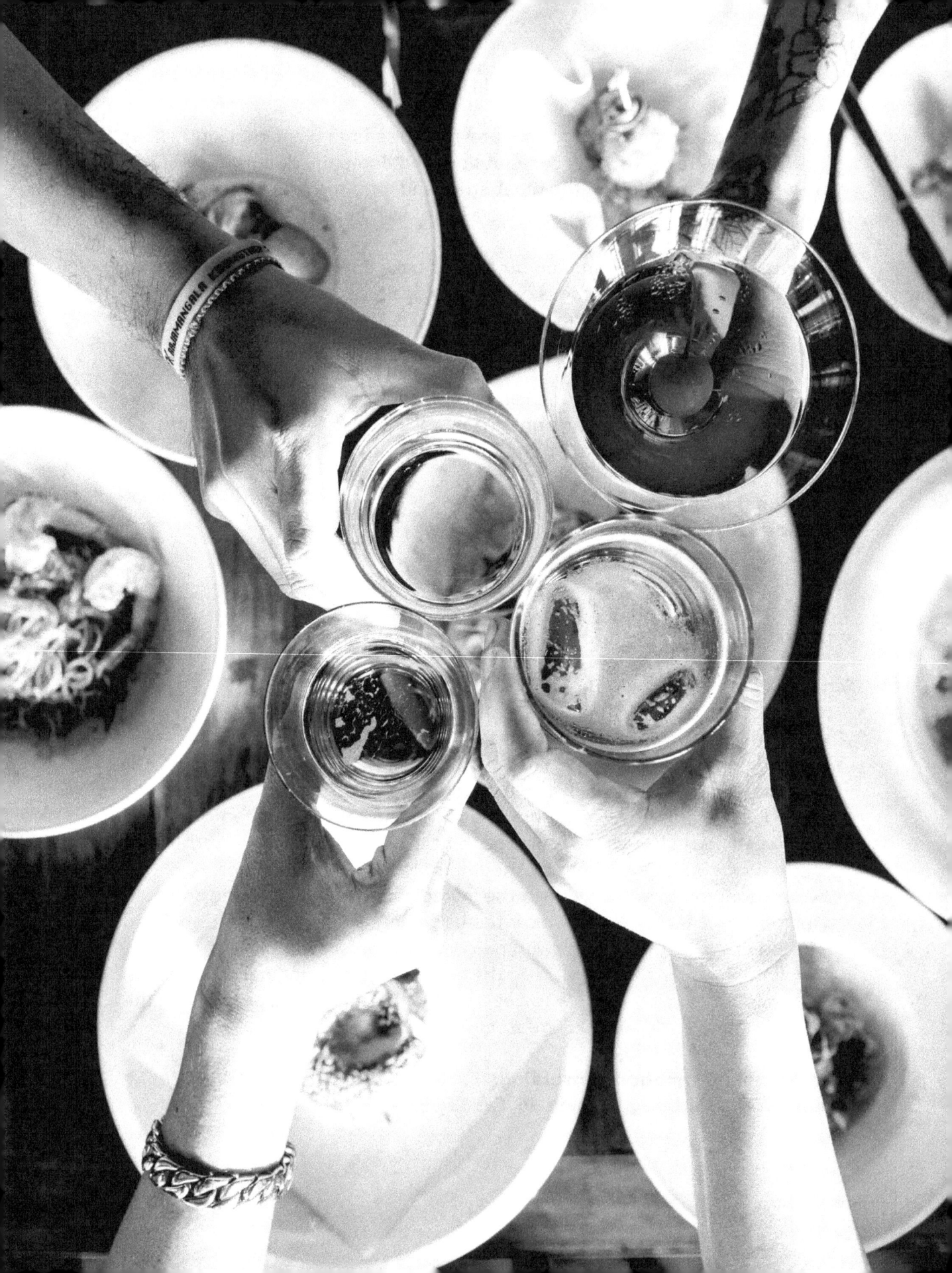

CHAPTER 7

KETO DIET
LUNCH RECIPES

SPICY BAKED CHICKEN

Serves 3   *Prep Time* 5 minutes   *Cook Time* 33 minutes   *Total Time* 38 minutes

Ingredients
- ✓ 1 pound boneless, skinless chicken breasts
- ✓ 1/4 teaspoon black pepper freshly ground
- ✓ 1/2 teaspoon sea salt
- ✓ 1/2 cup mild or spicy salsa
- ✓ 4 ounces cream cheese cut into large chunks
- ✓ 1 teaspoon parsley finely, chopped

Directions
1. Preheat your oven to 350 degrees F. Add the salsa and cream cheese to a heavy-weight cooking pan.
2. Put the saucepan over low heat and cook, stirring now and again until the cheese melts and fully mixes with the salsa. Season with salt and pepper and remove the mixture from heat.
3. Layer the skinless meat on a baking dish and add in the cheese and salsa mixture on top, to fully cover the breast.
4. Bake the mixture until the center of the chicken meat indicates 180 degrees on the meat thermometer, or for about 40 to 45 minutes.
5. Remove from the oven and top with fresh parsley. You can serve immediately or keep the chicken in the fridge in airtight containers. Please note that cooked chicken meat may hardly last beyond a week even when frozen.

Nutritional information per serving:
Calories: 291, Carbs 4g, Protein 34g, Fat 17g

CRISPY BAKED FISH STICKS

Serves 4 *Prep Time: 10 minutes* *Cook Time: 15 minutes* *Total Time: 25 minutes*

Ingredients

- ✓ 1 teaspoon water
- ✓ 1 large egg
- ✓ 1 (3.5-ounce) bag pork rinds
- ✓ 1 1/2 tablespoons coconut flour
- ✓ 12 ounces fresh cod fillets

Nutritional information per serving:
Calories 270, Carbs 1g, Protein 38g, Fat 11.5g

Directions

1. Preheat your oven to 400 degrees F. Meanwhile cut the cod fillets into strips, and season them with some salt and pepper.
2. Sprinkle the cod fillets with coconut flour then toss to fully cover. Put the pork rinds in a Zip top freezer bag and crush them into crumbs.
3. Once done, whisk the egg and water together and then dip each of the cod sticks into the egg mixture, and into the pork crumbs and put them in a greased baking sheet.
5. Bake until golden brown, or for 12 to 15 minutes, and serve immediately with some sauce and vegetables

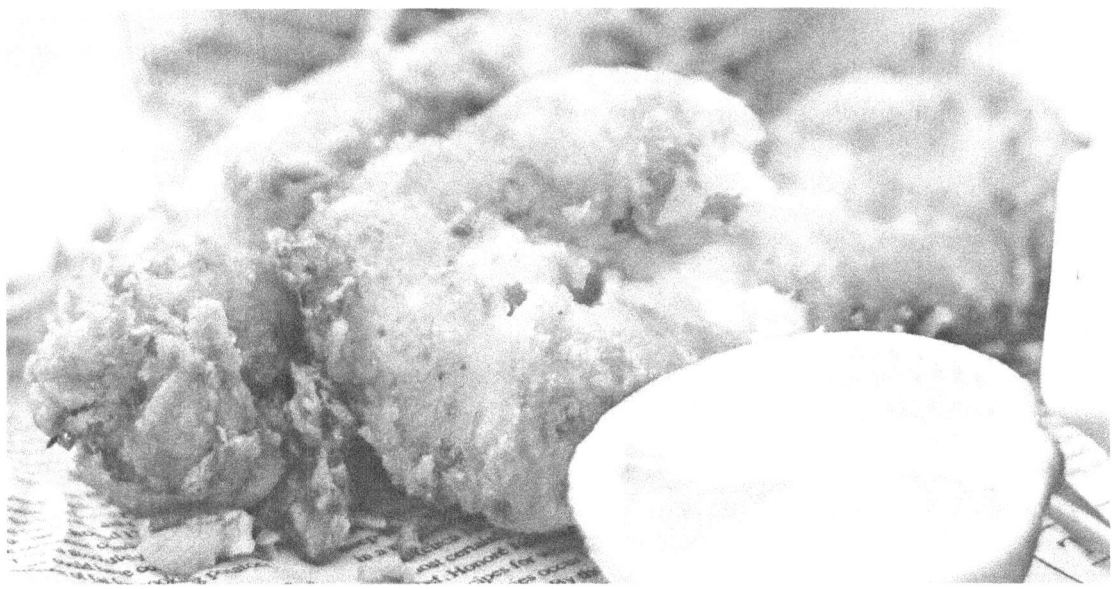

STIR FRY KIMCHI & PORK BELLY

Serves: 3 *Prep Time:* 5 minutes *Cook Time:* 15 minutes
Marinating Time: 10 minutes *Total Time:* 20 minutes

Ingredients
✓ 1 tablespoon sesame seeds
✓ 1 stalk green onion
✓ 1 lb. kimchi
✓ 1 tablespoon naturally-brewed rice wine
✓ 1 tablespoon naturally-brewed tamari
✓ 300g naturally raised pork belly

Directions
1. Begin by thinly slicing the pork belly and then marinate the meat in rice wine and naturally brewed tamari for around 10 minutes. Cut the kimchi into 1 inch size if it isn't precut.
2. Heat a heavy pan and then add in the marinated pork belly into the hot pan. Stir fry the pork for 5 to 10 minutes or until nicely browned.
3. Add in the cut kimchi into the pan and cook for 2 minutes, to fully blend pork and kimchi flavors.
4. Switch of the heat and slice the onion. Add it to the stir-fry, sprinkle with sesame seeds and serve.

Nutritional information per serving:
Calories 578, Carbs 6g, Protein 13.7g, Fat 33.82g

BACON WRAPPED PORK CHOPS

***Serves** 4-6* ***Prep Time:** 10 minutes* ***Cook Time:** 30 minutes* ***Total Time:** 40 minutes*

Ingredients
- ✓ 6 to 8 boneless pork chops
- ✓ 12 ounce bacon package (or larger if required)
- ✓ Fresh peppercorn grinder

Directions

1. Preheat your oven to 350 degrees F. Meanwhile place the chops on a plate, and season with fresh pepper.
2. Wrap individual pork chop in the raw bacon slices.
3. Grind a little more pepper over the meat-wrapped chops.
4. Put the prepared chops in a pan and bake them, flipping them after 15 minutes, for approximately 30 minutes.
5. Serve the bacon-wrapped pork chops while hot.

Nutritional information per serving:
Calories 513, Carbs 1g, Protein 51g, Fat 34g

SEARED TUNA STEAK

Serves 2   ***Prep Time:*** *15 minutes*   ***Cook Time:*** *6 minutes*   ***Total Time:*** *21 minutes*

Ingredients
- ✓ 1 teaspoon sesame seeds
- ✓ 1 tablespoon sesame oil
- ✓ 2 tablespoons soy sauce
- ✓ 2 (6-ounce) ahi tuna steaks
- ✓ Salt and pepper

Directions
1. Sprinkle salt and pepper on your tuna steaks and put them in a shallow bowl.
2. Whisk together sesame oil and soy sauce and then pour over the seasoned tuna steaks. Turn to coat then let them marinate for approximately 15 minutes.
3. Meanwhile over medium high heat, heat a large skillet until it is very hot.
4. Add in the steaks and cook until cooked through, or for around 3 minutes. Flip and let the tuna cook for another 2 or 3 minutes.
5. Slice the tuna about half-inch slices then serve garnished with sesame seeds.

Nutritional information per serving: Calories 255, Carbs 1g, Protein 40.5g, Fat 9g

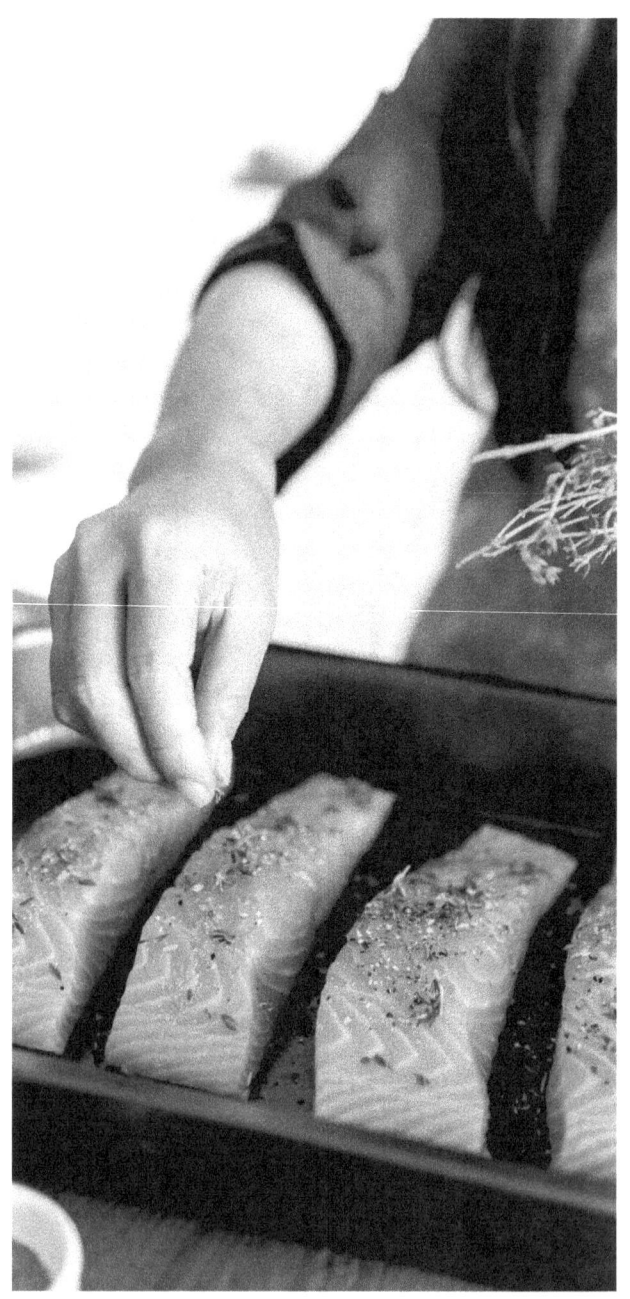

GARLIC BUTTER STEAK

Serves: *4*   ***Prep Time*** *10 minutes*   ***Cook Time*** *5 minutes*   ***Total Time*** *15 minutes*

Ingredients

- ✓ 1 tablespoon fresh flat-leaf parsley, chopped
- ✓ 4 tablespoons unsalted butter
- ✓ 2 tablespoons canola oil or vegetable oil
- ✓ Black pepper, freshly ground
- ✓ 1-1/2 pounds skirt steak, trimmed and cut into 4 pieces
- ✓ Kosher salt
- ✓ 6 medium cloves garlic

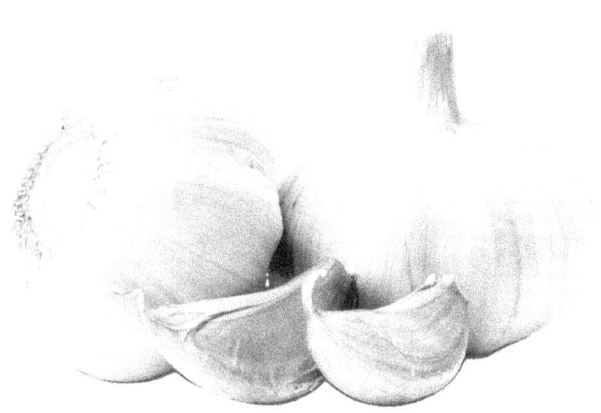

Directions

1. Peel the garlic cloves and then smash them using the side of a knife. prinkle with some salt and then mince the clove.
2. Pat dry the steak and season with salt and pepper on both sides. Over medium heat, heat oil in a 12-inch heavy-duty skillet.
3. Once the oil is shimmering hot, add in the seasoned steak and brown for about 2 to 3 minutes on each side.
4. Transfer the steak to a plate and let it cool until you are done with making the garlic butter.
5. Meanwhile, melt butter in an 8-inch skillet over low heat. Add in garlic and cook for 4 minutes as you swirl the pan a number of times.
6. Once lightly golden, add some salt to taste. Slice the steak and divide among 4 plates.
7. To serve, spoon garlic butter over the steak and sprinkle with chopped parsley.

Nutritional information per serving:
Calories 429, Carbs 2g, Protein 37g, Fat 31g

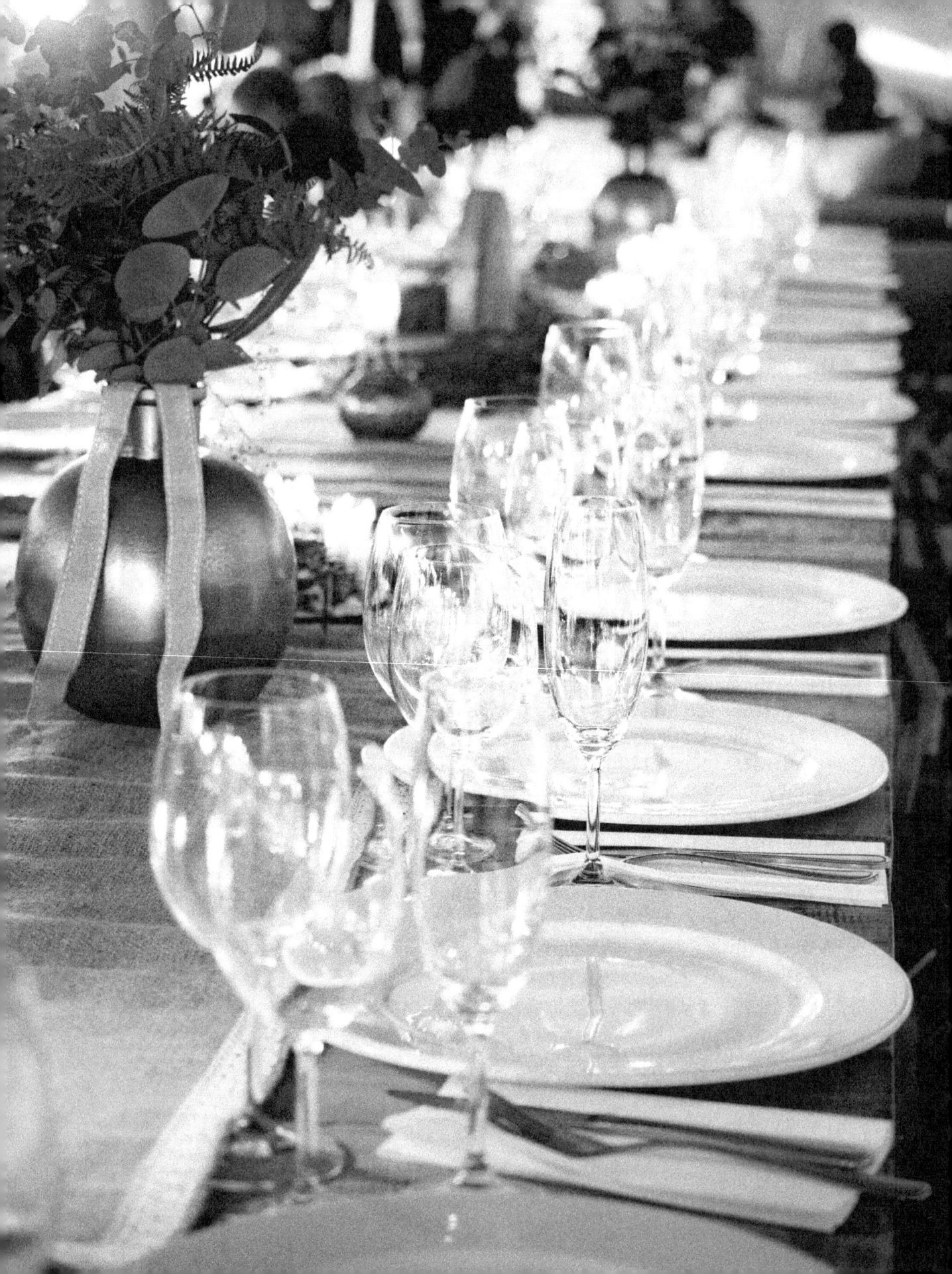

CHAPTER 8

KETO DIET
DINNER RECIPES

LEMON PEPPER SHEET PAN SALMON

Serves 4   *Prep Time:* 15 minutes   *Cook Time:* 15 minutes   *Total Time:* 30 minutes

Ingredients

- ✓ 1 1/2 tablespoons lemon herb seasoning (1 teaspoon thyme leaves, 2 teaspoons oregano, 2 teaspoons basil, ½ teaspoon salt, 2 tablespoons lemon pepper)
- ✓ 1 tablespoon olive oil
- ✓ 1 lemon sliced into rounds
- ✓ 1 bunch asparagus ends trimmed
- ✓ 12 oz green beans ends trimmed
- ✓ 16 oz salmon cut into four portions
- ✓ Lemon Dill Yogurt
- ✓ 1 tablespoon lemon zest
- ✓ 1/2 teaspoon dill
- ✓ 1/4 teaspoon salt
- ✓ 1 clove garlic minced
- ✓ 3/4 cup yogurt

Directions

1. Preheat your oven to 425 degrees F.
2. Meanwhile, toss asparagus and green beans with a tablespoon of the lemon seasoning and olive oil.
3. Arrange the mixture on two sheets of papers or one large sheet along with some lemon slices.
4. Add in the fish fillets and sprinkle with the rest of the herb seasoning. Layer a few lemon slices on the salmon fillets.
5. Bake until the fillets are cooked through, or for approximately 12 to 15 minutes.
6. Stir together the ingredients for the lemon dill yogurt then spoon the mixture over the salmon fillets and vegetables.
7. In case you want to prep ahead, you can chop the veggies and keep them in an airtight container along with the lemon slices. Toss them with the herb seasoning and olive oil and store for a maximum of 3 days.
8. You can also keep the salmon fillets in the fridge while seasoned with the herb seasoning for about 2-3 days.
9. Stir together the ingredients for lemon dill yogurt and keep in the fridge for not more than 7 days.
10. You can make the dish ahead and store it in the fridge about 3 days prior to cooking.
11. Once ready to cook, just spread all ingredients on a sheet pan and cook for approximately 12 to 15 minutes.

Nutritional information per serving:
Calories: 201, Carbs: 10g, Protein: 25g, Fat: 6g

BAKED MEATBALLS

Serves 3 **Prep Time:** *10 minutes* **Cook Time:** *20 minutes* **Total Time:** *30 minutes*

Ingredients

- ✓ 1/4 cup fresh rosemary, roughly chopped
- ✓ 2 garlic cloves, minced
- ✓ 1/2 medium yellow onion, minced
- ✓ 1 teaspoon salt
- ✓ 1/2 teaspoon pepper
- ✓ 1 tablespoon apple cider vinegar
- ✓ 2 tablespoons grass-fed ghee
- ✓ 1 1/4 pounds pastured ground beef
- ✓ Optional:
- ✓ 1 teaspoon crushed red pepper flakes

Directions

1. Preheat your oven to 350 degrees F. Meanwhile add all ingredients into a mixing bowl and combine with your hands.
2. Once mixed, set aside, and line a baking tray with parchment papers.
3. Roll the dough mixture into small balls, with about 1 tablespoon of mixture per each meat ball.
4. As soon as you are done with rolling, put them on the parchment lined baking tray and bake until cooked through, or for approximately 20 minutes.
5. Serve the meatballs warm with some vegetables or let them cool and store them in an airtight container in the freezer or refrigerator.

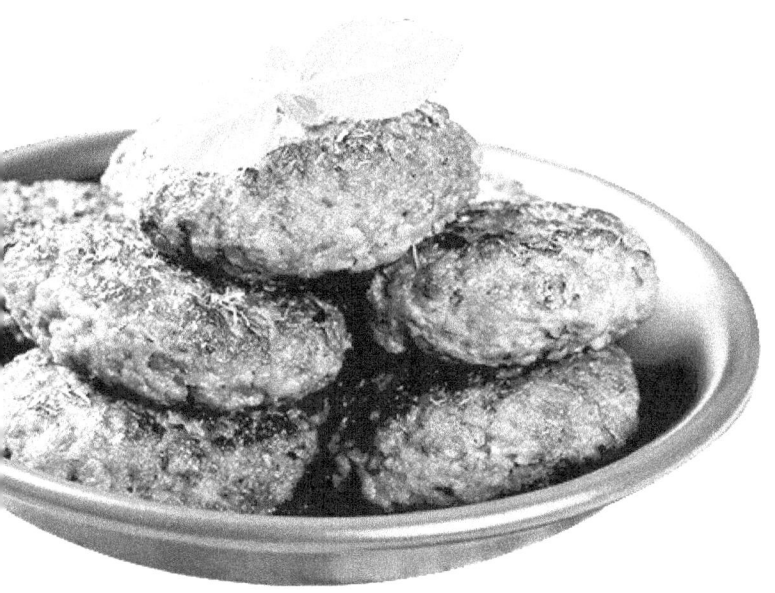

Nutritional information per serving:
Calories: 474, Carbs: 5.6g, Protein: 61.3g, Fat: 21.7g

LOW CARB CHICKEN SKILLET

Serves 4   *Prep Time* 15 minutes   *Cook Time* 10 minutes   *Total Time* 25 minutes

Ingredients

- ✓ 1 1/2 cups green beans
- ✓ 1/2 head riced cauliflower, about 4 cups
- ✓ 1/4 cup tomato sauce
- ✓ 1/2 teaspoon salt
- ✓ 1/2 teaspoon garam masala
- ✓ 1/2 teaspoon ground coriander
- ✓ 1/2 teaspoon garlic powder
- ✓ 1/2 teaspoon onion powder
- ✓ 1 teaspoon curry powder
- ✓ 1 teaspoon cumin
- ✓ 1/4 cup water
- ✓ Salt & pepper
- ✓ 1 lb boneless skinless chicken thighs
- ✓ 1 tablespoon olive oil

To serve
Plain yogurt, optional

Directions

1. Heat a large pan, and add in the chicken. Cook until cooked through, or for approximately 5 minutes each side.
2. Transfer the cooked meat to a clean plate and then drain any excess oil. Add water into the pan and the spices, and simmer while stirring continuously for about 2 minutes.
3. Add in the tomato sauce and stir until fully blended with the spices.
4. Add in the riced cauliflower preferably in two batches. Stir the mixture until the tomato sauce and spices have incorporated.
5. Add in green beans and cook until cooked through, or for around 2 to 4 minutes.
6. You can serve immediately or store in sealed containers for up to 4 days. To serve, just reheat until very hot.

Nutritional information per serving:
Calories: 207, Carbs 8g, Protein: 24g, Fat: 8g

CHICKEN WITH CAULIFLOWER RICE

Serves 4   Prep Time: 20 minutes   Cook Time: 30 minutes   Total Time: 50 minutes

Ingredients

For the Chicken
- ✓ 1/2 teaspoon honey
- ✓ 1/8 teaspoon sea salt
- ✓ 2 teaspoons minced garlic
- ✓ 1/3 cup fresh cilantro, chopped
- ✓ 1/4 cup lime juice
- ✓ Salt and pepper
- ✓ 2 tablespoons olive oil
- ✓ 1 lb. boneless, skinless chicken breast

For the Cauliflower Rice
- ✓ 1/4 cup red onion, raw
- ✓ 1/8 sea salt
- ✓ 1 teaspoon ground cumin
- ✓ 2 teaspoons garlic powder
- ✓ 3 cups cauliflower rice
- ✓ 2 tablespoons olive oil

For the Bowls
- ✓ 1 avocado, chopped
- ✓ 1 cup cherry tomatoes, halved

Directions

1. Over medium heat, heat the olive oil in a pan until bubbling hot. Add in the chicken and then cook for about 5 to 8 minutes each side.
2. Allow the chicken to cool down for around 15 minutes, and then slice it; set aside.
3. Add in the remaining ingredients for the chicken into a bowl large enough to accommodate them. Combine well.
4. Put the sliced chicken in a bowl and toss with the dressing. Keep refrigerated.
5. To make the cauliflower rice, add some olive oil into a large skillet and heat over medium heat for around 5 minutes.
6. Add in red onions and cook.
7. Serve or instead keep in the fridge for not more than 4 days.
8. To serve, just put the chicken, cooked cauliflower rice, 1/4 of an avocado and 1/4 cup of the tomatoes in a bowl and serve.

Nutritional information per serving:
Calories 378, Carbs 16g, Protein 32g, Fat 21g

RANCH CHICKEN JAR SALADS

Serves 4   *Prep Time* 20 minutes   *Cook Time* 7 minutes   *Total Time* 27 minutes

Ingredients

- ✓ 1 cup mozzarella, shredded
- ✓ 1 bell pepper, chopped into small pieces
- ✓ 1 cup cucumbers, cut into rounds
- ✓ 1 cup cherry tomatoes
- ✓ 4 cups romaine lettuce, cut into bite-sized pieces
- ✓ 1/2 cup homemade ranch dressing
- ✓ Salt & pepper
- ✓ 1 lb boneless skinless chicken breast
- ✓ 1 tablespoon olive oil

Directions

1. Heat olive oil in a large non-stick pan over medium heat.
2. Add in chicken and season with salt and pepper. Cook until cooked through and no longer pink or for about 5 to 7 minutes.
3. Meanwhile stir the half-cup homemade ranch dressings and add 2 tablespoons of the dressing to the bottom of 4 mason jars.
4. Add cooked chicken in the bottom of mason jars, then bell peppers, mozzarella cheese, tomatoes and cucumbers.
5. Press the romaine lettuce at the top of the jar and seal well. Store the mason jar in the fridge for up to 4 days.
6. To serve just shake the jar and pour the contents into a bowl or just shake the jar up and eat right out of the jar if large enough.

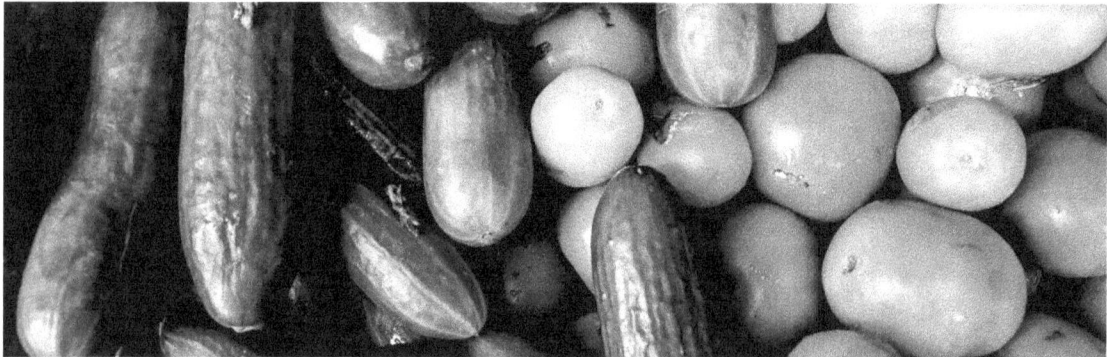

Nutritional information per serving:
Calories: 417, Carbs: 8g, Protein: 32g, Fat: 28g

CHEESY CHICKEN AND RICE MEAL PREP

Serves 4   *Prep Time* 20 minutes   *Cook Time* 20 minutes   *Total Time* 40 minutes

Ingredients
✓ 1 cup shredded mozzarella cheese
✓ 1 crown broccoli or 4 cups of bite-sized pieces
✓ Salt and pepper
✓ 2 tablespoons olive oil
✓ 1/2 head cauliflower

For Chicken
✓ 1/4 teaspoon pepper
✓ 1/4 teaspoon salt
✓ 1 teaspoon onion powder
✓ 1 teaspoon garlic powder
✓ 1 tablespoon olive oil
✓ 1 lb boneless skinless chicken breasts

Directions
1. Begin by making the cauliflower rice. Just cut the cauliflower into equally sized pieces and then pulse in the food processor until well broken down into rice, or for 10 to 15 times.
2. Into a non-stick pan, add in a tablespoon of olive oil and then heat the oil over medium heat.
3. Add in the riced cauliflower and cook until softened, or for about 5 minutes or so.
4. Season the rice with salt and pepper and then distribute the cauliflower among 4 two-cup capacity containers.
5. Into the same pan, add a tablespoon of olive oil along with broccoli. Cook until the broccoli is slightly softened, or for about 5 to 7 minutes.
6. Now add the softened broccoli to the four containers that have riced cauliflower.
7. Toss the chicken with garlic powder, olive oil, pepper, onion powder and salt.
8. Cook the seasoned chicken over medium heat for about 5 to 7 minutes, or until cooked through.
9. Add the chicken into the containers. Distribute the shredded mozzarella between the storage containers and keep in the fridge for a maximum of 4 days.
10. To serve just heat in the microwave until hot, stir to blend and then enjoy.

Nutritional information per serving:
Calories: 329, Carbs: 5g, Protein: 31g, Fat: 19g

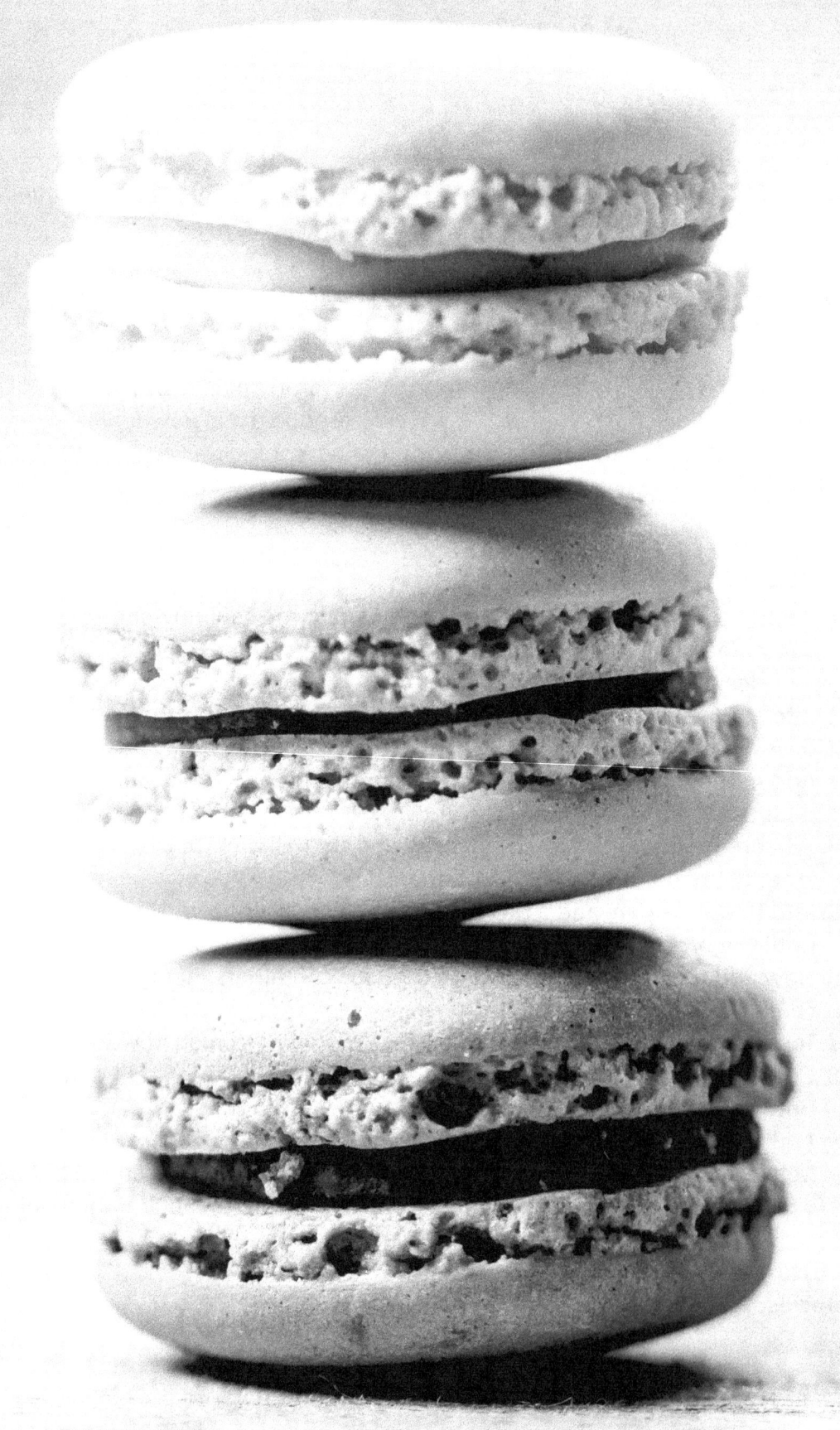

CHAPTER 9

KETO DIET SNACKS

BLACKBERRY NUT FAT BOMBS

Serves: 12 *Prep time:* 20 minutes *Cook time:* 10 minutes *Total time:* 30 minutes

Ingredients
- ✓ 1/2 teaspoon lemon juice
- ✓ 1/2 teaspoon vanilla extract
- ✓ 1 cup coconut butter
- ✓ 1 cup coconut oil
- ✓ 3 tablespoons mascarpone cheese
- ✓ 1 cup blackberries
- ✓ 4 oz. cream cheese
- ✓ 2 oz. macadamia nuts, crushed
Stevia to taste

Directions
1. Crush the nuts and then press them into the bottom of a mold or baking dish.
2. Bake the nuts in a preheated oven at 325 degree F until cooked through or golden brown.
3. Once done, remove from the oven and let it cool. Spread a layer of cream cheese over the nuts.
4. In a bowl, mix lemon juice, vanilla, coconut butter, coconut oil, mascarpone cheese and blackberries until smooth.
5. Pour the well-blended mixture over the cream cheese and keep frozen for 30-60 minutes.
6. Finally remove from the freezer and store in the refrigerator until ready to serve.

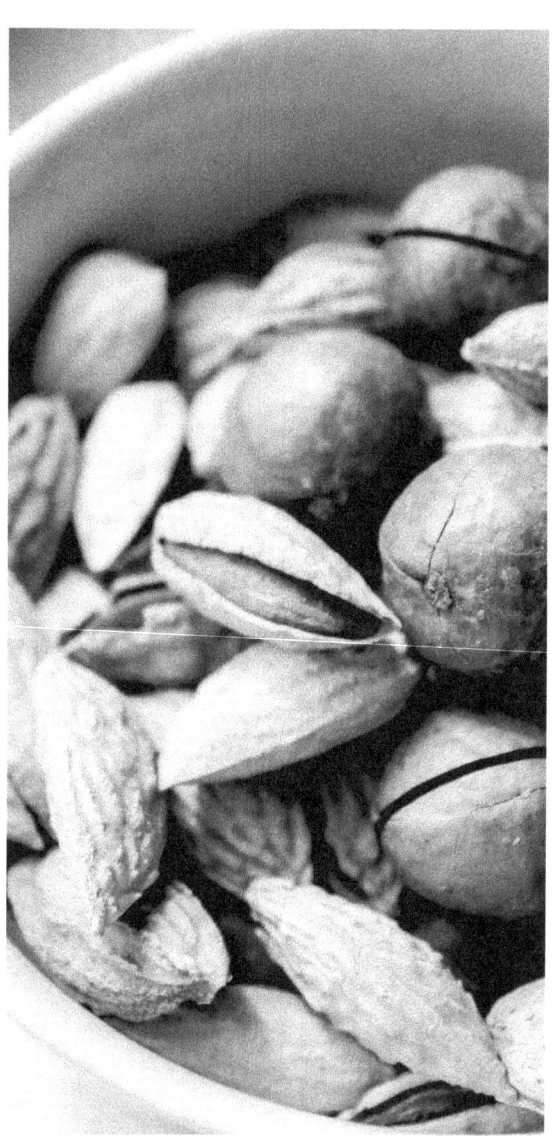

Nutritional information per serving: Calories392, Carb 2g, Protein 4g, Fat 50g

SALMON AND CREAM CHEESE BITES

Serves 4 **Prep Time** 10 minutes   **Cook Time** 10 minutes   **Total Time** 20 minutes

Ingredients
- ✓ 1.8 oz cream cheese
- ✓ 1 teaspoon dried dill
- ✓ 1.8 oz fresh or smoked salmon slices
- ✓ 1.8 oz shredded/grated cheese
- ✓ 1/2 teaspoon salt
- ✓ 1 cup coconut milk or coconut cream
- ✓ 6 medium sized eggs

Directions
1. Into a large pouring jug, whisk together eggs, coconut milk and salt and then fold in dill, smoked salmon, grated cheese and chopped cream cheese.
2. Pour the batter into greased silicon molds or mini muffin trays. Bake the mixture at about 350 degrees F for about 10 to 15 minutes.
3. Allow to cool before serving.

Nutritional information per serving:
Calories 44, Carbs 0.1g, Protein 1g, Fat 4g

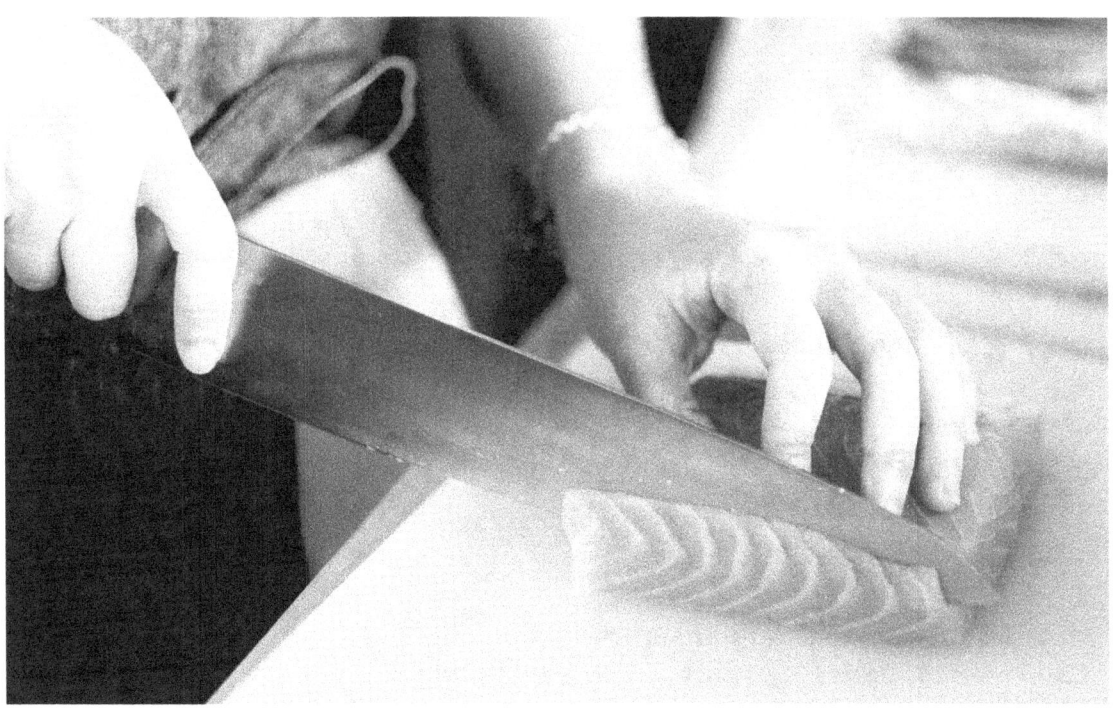

GREEN TEA MUG CAKE

Serves 2   ***Prep Time:** 5 minutes*   ***Total Time:** 7 minutes*

Ingredients
- ✓ 1 ounce coconut milk
- ✓ 1 teaspoon erythritol
- ✓ 1 teaspoon baking powder
- ✓ 4 tablespoons almond flour
- ✓ 2 tablespoons green tea protein powder
- ✓ 1 large Egg

Directions
1. Combine all the dry ingredients in a small bowl.
2. Mix the wet ingredients in the same bowl, and mix using a hand mixer or a fork.
3. Pour the batter into a small bowl or mug and microwave until cooked through, or for 1 to 2 minutes.
4. You can serve or keep it for a few days.

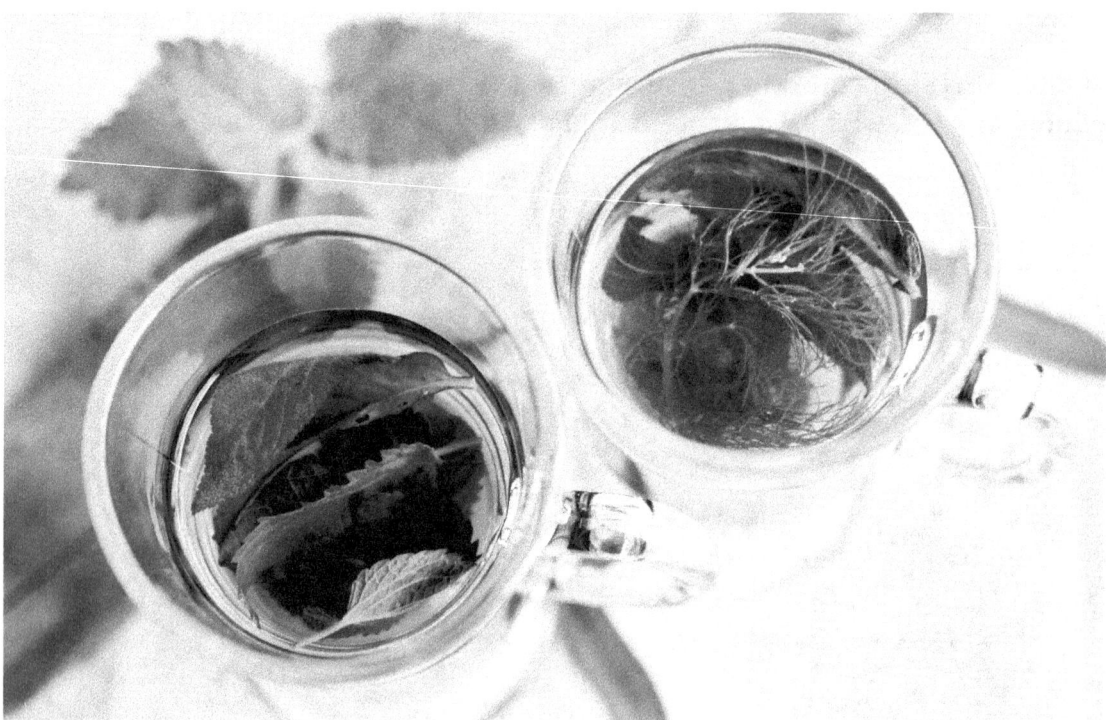

Nutritional information per serving:
Calories 321, Carbs 1g, Protein 24g, Fat 23.7g

KETO HOAGIE BISCUITS

Serves 12 **Prep Time:** *5 minutes* **Cook Time:** *25 minutes* **Passive Time:** *25 minutes*

Ingredients
- ✓ 1 cup pepperoni or ham, chopped
- ✓ 1 cup provolone cheese, shredded
- ✓ 1 & ¼ cups blanched almond flour
- ✓ 1 packet Italian dressing mix
- ✓ ¼ cup filtered water
- ✓ ¼ cup organic heavy cream
- ✓ 1 large egg (organic, pasture raised)
- ✓ 4 ounces organic cultured cream cheese

Directions
1. Preheat your oven to 350 degrees F, and then grease a muffin pan.
2. Mix heavy cream, water, egg, cream cheese and Italian dressing in a blender until smooth.
3. Add in almond flour into the mixture and mix well blended.
4. Fold in the ham or pepperoni and distribute the batter among 12 muffin cups.
5. Bake for approximately 20 minutes.
6. Let it cool down in the pan for around 5 minutes or so and then transfer to a cooling rack.
7. Serve the biscuit either warm or chilled.

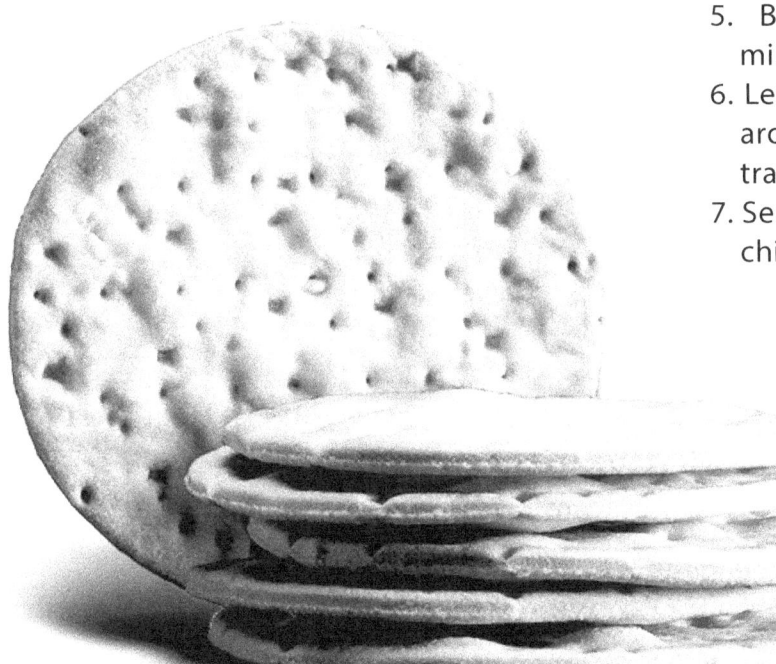

Nutritional information per serving:
Calories 249, Carbs 6g, Protein 11g, Fat 21g

SUGAR FREE COCONUT BALLS

Serves 12   ***Prep Time*** *40 minutes*   ***Total Time*** *40 minutes*

Ingredients
- ✓ Stevia powder to taste
- ✓ 1/2 tsp ground cinnamon
- ✓ 1 cup shredded coconut, unsweetened
- ✓ 1 cup coconut butter

Directions
1. Put coconut butter, stevia and cinnamon in a glass bowl and set it over a double boiler.
2. Heat the mixture to melt, mix the ingredients and then place the mixture in the fridge for approximately 20 minutes.
3. Once this time is up, remove from the fridge and roll into about 12 balls.
4. Put the balls in the fridge and allow them to set for another 20 minutes.
5. Put some shredded coconut flakes on a plate and roll the coconut balls over.
6. Keep the balls in the fridge for up to 14 days.

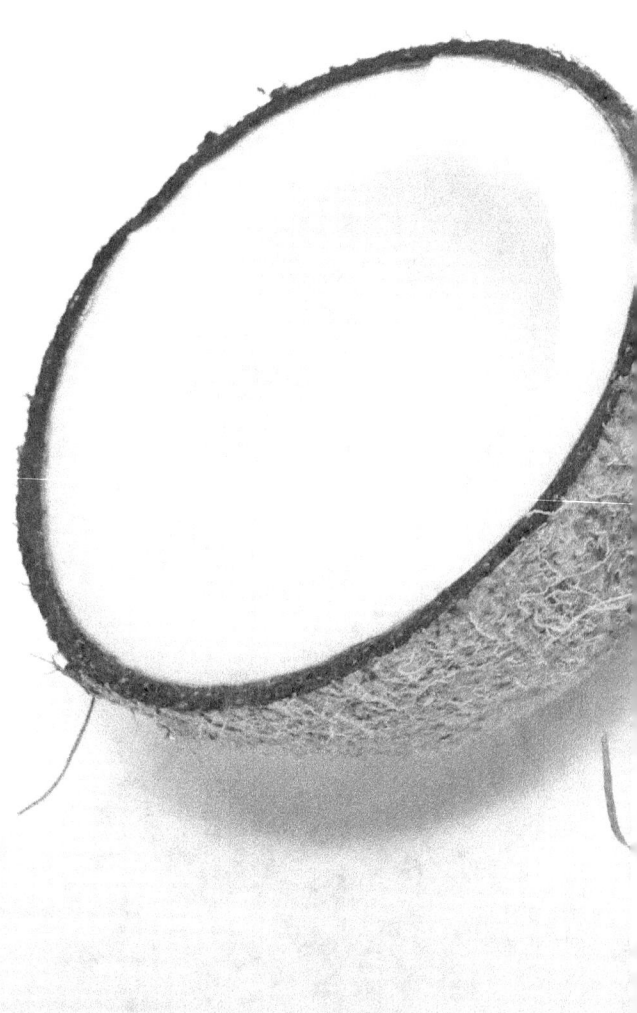

Nutritional information per serving:
Calories 196, Carbs 6g, Protein 2g, Fat 18g

COCONUT CRACK BARS

Serves 20   ***Prep Time:*** *2 minutes*   ***Cook Time:*** *3 minutes*   ***Total Time:*** *5 minutes*

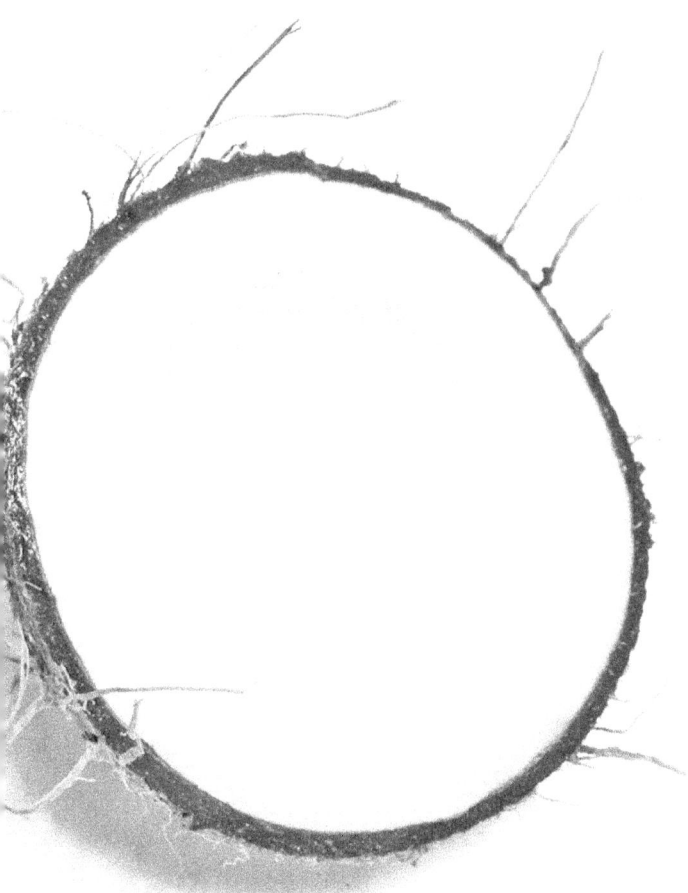

Ingredients

✓ 1/4 cup monk fruit sweetened maple syrup
✓ 1 cup coconut oil, melted
✓ 3 cups Shredded coconut flakes, unsweetened

Directions

1. Get a parchment paper and line an 8 by 8 inch pan, then set aside.
2. Add shredded coconut to a large mixing bowl and then add in maple syrup along with coconut oil.
3. Mix the ingredients until you obtain a thick batter. In case you find it too crumbly, consider adding some more syrup or a little amount of water.
4. Pour the crack bar mixture into the prepared pan and then wet your hands. Press the dough firmly in place.
5. Keep it refrigerated to help firm up. The bars should keep for a maximum of 7 days, while covered at room temperature and for 30 days while in the fridge. The bars can last up to 2 months in the freezer.

Nutritional information per serving: Calories 108, Carbs 2g, Protein 2g, Fat 11g

KETOGENIC FAT BALLS

Servings: 16   *Prep Time: 15 minutes*   *Total Time: 15 minutes*

Ingredients
- ✓ 1/4 teaspoon sea salt
- ✓ 1/2 teaspoon ground cinnamon
- ✓ 3 tablespoons cold water
- ✓ 1 teaspoon pure vanilla extract
- ✓ 2 tablespoons pure maple syrup, sugar free
- ✓ 1/2 cup coconut oil melted and cooled
- ✓ 2 scoops Vital Proteins Marine Collagen
- ✓ 1/4 cup cacao nibs, optional
- ✓ 1/3 cup nut or seed butter
- ✓ 1 cup shredded coconut, unsweetened
- ✓ 1.5 cups raw nuts

Directions
1. Add raw nuts to a blender or food processor and then blend until fine.
2. Add the rest of the ingredients in the food processor and blend until you have thick but sticky paste.
3. Now roll the dough into 16 or 20 equally sized balls.
4. Keep the balls refrigerated until ready to serve. As balls thaw quickly, keep them in the freezer instead.

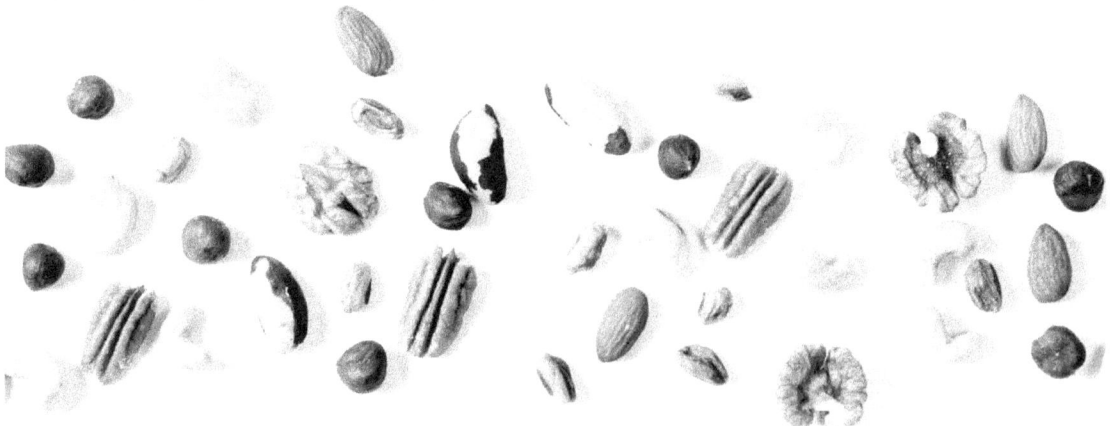

Nutritional information per serving:
Calories 249, Carbs 6g, Protein 11g, Fat 6g

CRISPY JALAPEÑO CHEESE CRACKERS

Serves 16   *Prep Time:* 10 minutes   *Cook Time:* 30 minutes   *Total Time:* 40 minutes

Ingredients
- ✓ 4 medium jalapeno peppers sliced
- ✓ 1 pound sliced cheese hot pepper or cheddar

Directions
1. Preheat your oven to 425 degrees F. Meanwhile get a silicon liner or parchment paper and line a baking sheet.
2. Cut the sliced cheddar into 1.5 inch squares and slice the jalapenos either thinly or thickly preferably using a mandolin.
3. Layer the slices of cheese about 1 inch apart on the lined baking sheet and top the cheese with a slice of jalapeno.
4. Bake for approximately 10 to 15 minutes in the middle of the oven. Be aware that cook time depends on how thick you slice the jalapenos and the type of baking sheet you are using.
5. Keep and remove from the oven as soon as its lightly brown. In case you're preparing multiple pans simultaneously, rotate the racks after every 3 minutes to facilitate even baking.
6. Remove the baking pan from the oven and let it cook for about 15 minutes, to crisp up.
7. Transfer to a cooling rack to cool fully and then store them in an airtight container for about 2 to 3 days.

Nutritional information per serving:
Calories 106, Carbs 1g, Protein 7g, Fat 9g

LOW CARB CAULIFLOWER PIZZA MUFFINS

Serves 12   **Prep Time** *20 minutes*   **Cook Time** *25 minutes*   **Total Time** *45 minutes*

Ingredients
- ✓ 1/2 cup shredded cheese for tops
- ✓ 3-4 sliced 12 teaspoons pizza sauce
- ✓ 1/2 teaspoon baking powder
- ✓ 3/4 cup almond flour
- ✓ 1 1/2 cups shredded cheese
- ✓ 1 teaspoon dried oregano
- ✓ 1 teaspoon dried basil
- ✓ 1/2 teaspoon salt
- ✓ 3 large eggs
- ✓ 3 cups riced cauliflower

Directions
1. Preheat your oven to 350 degrees F. Meanwhile line a muffin tray with silicon liners or parchment paper. Alternatively coat it with cooking spray.
2. Stir together cheddar cheese, oregano, basil, eggs, cauliflower, baking powder and almond flour in a large bowl.
3. Distribute the batter between 12 muffin cups. Top each of the muffins with a few slices of pepperoni, a teaspoon of pizza sauce and some shredded cheese.
4. Bake until cooked through, or for approximately 25 to 28 minutes.
5. Serve or keep frozen in the fridge for about 3 to 4 days preferably in a sealed container.
6. To last longer, keep them frozen in the freezer for a maximum of 3 months! Just wrap individual muffin in plastic and keep in a storage container or a large bag.
7. To serve, simply heat in the microwave until the cheese has melted and is bubbly. You can serve either hot or cold.

Nutritional information per serving:
Calories 164, Carbs 4g, Protein 9g, Fat 12g

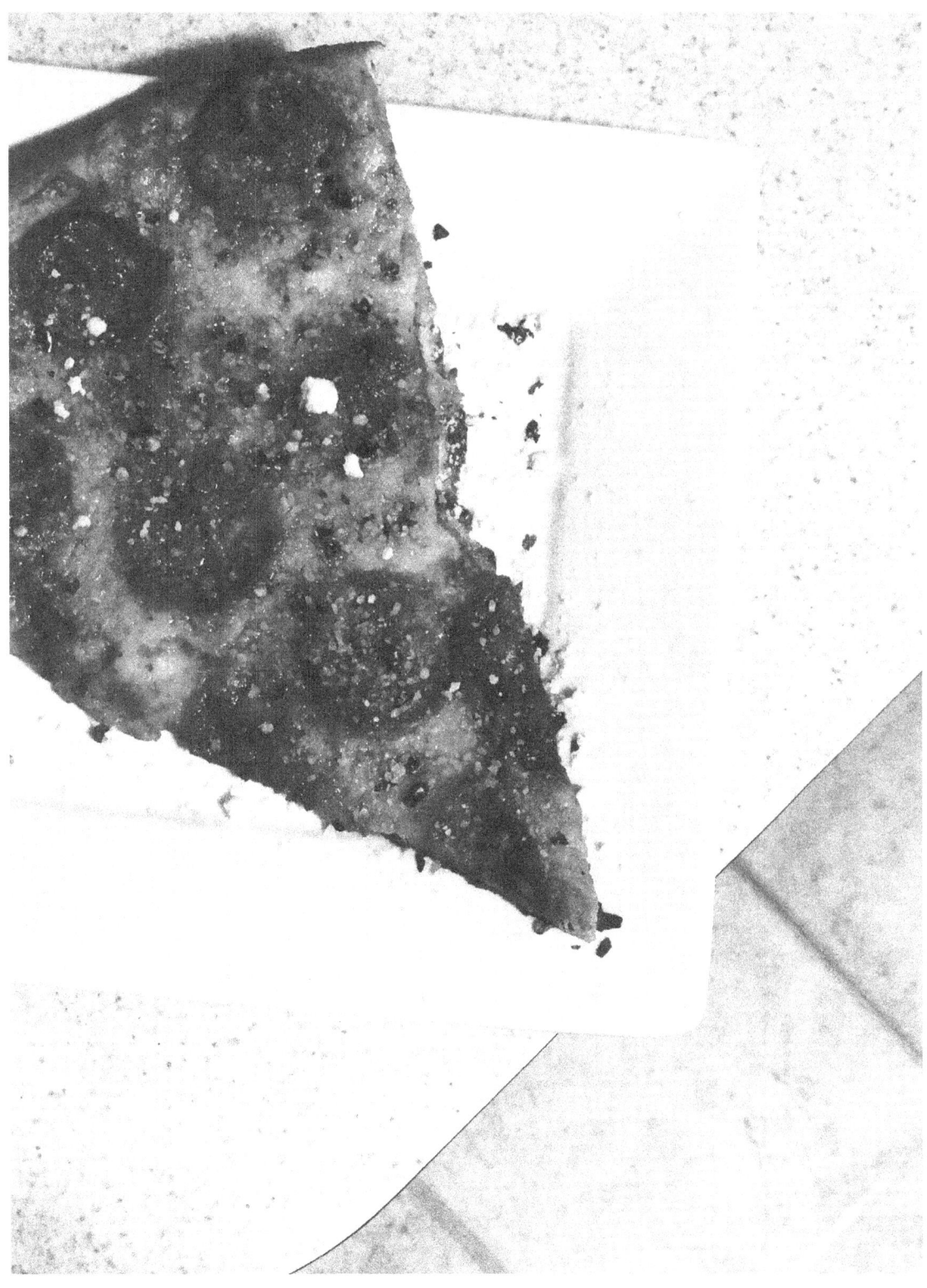

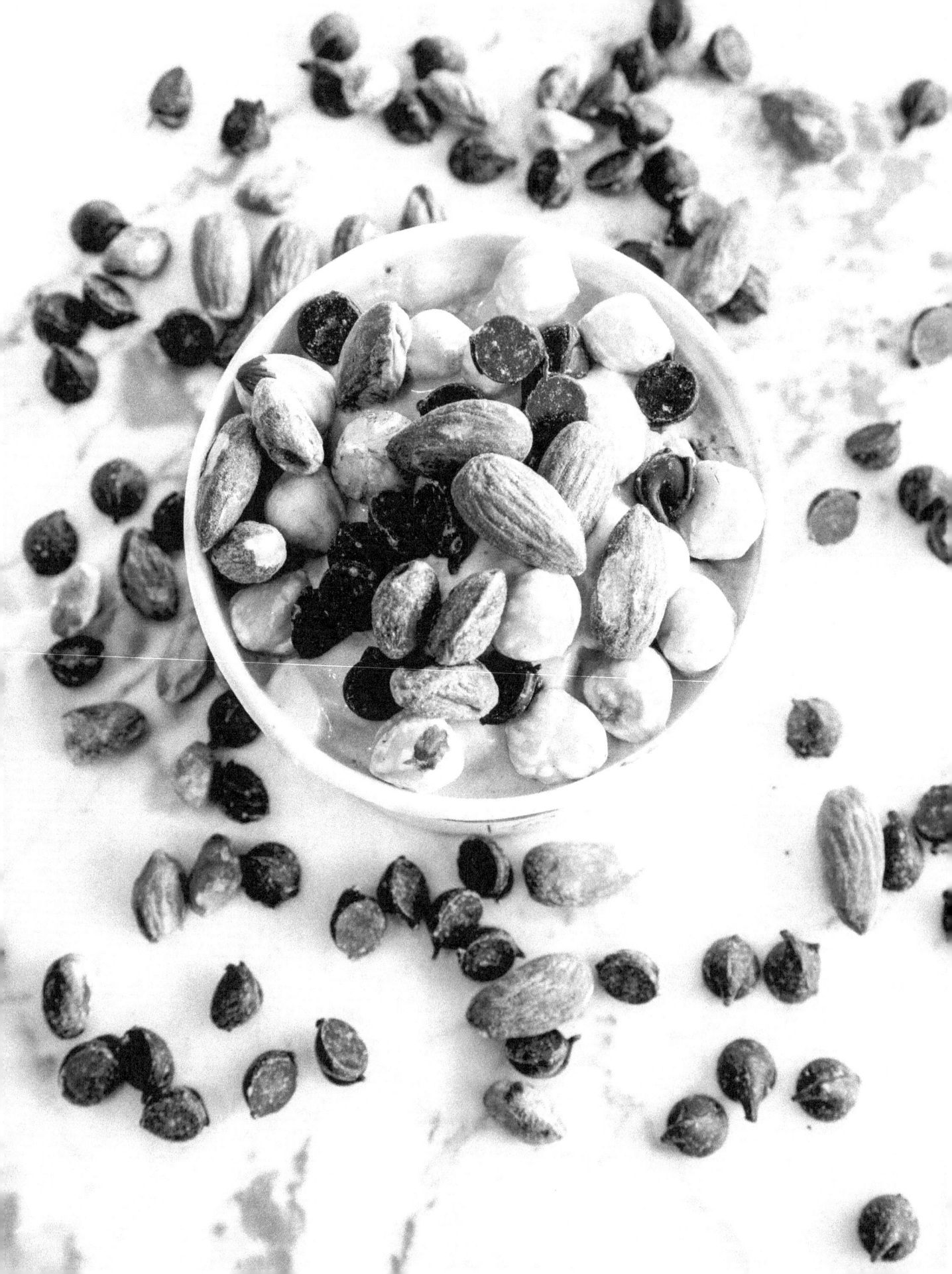

CONCLUSION

Indeed, the keto diet offers so many benefits you do not want to miss out on. The most important thing to bear in mind is to keep your carb intake below 20 grams/day when you are on a keto diet. It is the very low levels of carbs that will help keep your body in ketosis.

Remember that when your body is in ketosis, the body can switch from using carbs as the primary energy source to using ketones instead. This way, you get an opportunity to tap into incredible energy reserves, boost your moods, burn excess fats, lose weight, and keep your shape in check!

Once you realize your health and weight loss goals, you can choose to keep going with keto or add in small amounts of carbs into your diet. The most important thing is to ensure that you adopt a diet plan that ensure your weight and overall health stays in check.

Trust me; you will never regret choosing embarking on a keto diet journey!

If you found the book valuable, kindly recommend it to others? One way to do that is to post a review on Amazon.

Click here to leave a review on amazon.com

Or use this link on your computer: https://amzn.to/2yxt1uO

So, what is it going to be for you for the rest of 2019? Choose the keto diet today and get the shape you have been dreaming of all these years. Plus, you get to enjoy a healthy body.

If you require any further information, feel free to contact me: contact@alphaketo.net

Good luck!

www.ingramcontent.com/pod-product-compliance
Lightning Source LLC
Chambersburg PA
CBHW080851220526
45467CB00008B/2470